THE EASY WAY TO BETTER SLEEP

How to free yourself from sleepless nights

ALLEN CARR

with
JOHN DICEY

SIRIUS

To Sue Bolshaw, Paul Baker, Monique Douglas, Joan Halley, Indi Flahive-Gilbert, Colleen Dwyer and Chris Pitt – heroes of our global HQ team.

SIRIUS

This edition published in 2023 by Sirius Publishing, a division of Arcturus Publishing Limited, 26/27 Bickels Yard, 151–153 Bermondsey Street, London SE1 3HA

ISBN: 978-1-3988-1742-5
AD010571US

Printed in the US

This book is not intended to take the place of advice from a trained medical professional.

ALLEN CARR

Allen Carr was a chain-smoker for over 30 years. In 1983, after countless failed attempts to quit, he went from 100 cigarettes a day to zero without suffering withdrawal pangs, without using willpower and without putting on weight. He realized that he had discovered what the world had been waiting for—the easy way to stop smoking—and embarked on a mission to help cure the world's smokers.

As a result of the phenomenal success of his method, he gained an international reputation as the world's leading expert on stopping smoking and his network of centers now spans the globe. His first book, *Allen Carr's Easy Way to Stop Smoking*, remains a global bestseller and has been published in more than 40 different languages. Easyway books have now sold more than 20 million copies. Hundreds of thousands of smokers have successfully quit at Allen Carr's Easyway centers where, with a success rate of over 90 percent, they guarantee you'll find it easy to stop or your money back.

Allen Carr's Easyway method has been successfully applied to a host of issues including sleep, weight control, alcohol, and a dozen other addictions and fears. A list of Allen Carr centers appears at the back of this book. Should you require any assistance or if you have any questions, please do not hesitate to contact your nearest center.

For more information about Allen Carr's Easyway, please visit **www.AllenCarr.com**

Allen Carr's Easyway

The key that will set you free

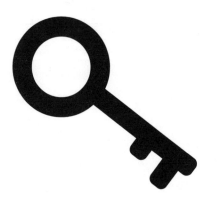

CONTENTS

IT'S ESSENTIAL THAT YOU DON'T SKIP THIS IMPORTANT
INTRODUCTION

BY JOHN DICEY, CO-FOUNDER, GLOBAL CEO AND SENIOR THERAPIST, ALLEN CARR'S EASYWAY

Welcome to *Allen Carr's Easy Way to Better Sleep*. Allen Carr's reputation in the field of addiction treatment and behavior change was built on his huge success in helping smokers to quit. His Easyway method was so successful that it quickly became, and remains, a global phenomenon. From the earliest days of Easyway, Allen was inundated with requests from sufferers of countless other addictions and issues, imploring him to expand his method to address their particular circumstances. By the turn of the century, Allen had assembled a team of bright, loyal, and dedicated senior therapists who went on to help him not only apply the method to all those addictions and issues but also play a key role in delivering Allen Carr's Easyway method across the globe.

The responsibility for ensuring that our books are faithful to Allen Carr's original method is mine, and it's an honor to be writing this important introduction. Rest assured, once you've read it, I'll leave you in Allen's capable hands. It has been suggested to me that I describe myself as the author of the books we've published since Allen passed away. In my view, that would be quite wrong.

That's because every new book is written strictly in accordance with Allen Carr's brilliant Easyway method. In our new books, we have merely updated the format to bring it up to date and make it as relevant as possible for the modern-day audience. There is not a word in our books that Allen didn't write or wouldn't have written if he were still with us and, for that reason, the updates, anecdotes, and analogies that are not his own work—that were contemporized or added by me—are written clearly in Allen's voice to seamlessly complement the original text and method.

I consider myself privileged to have worked closely with Allen on Easyway books while he was still alive, gaining insight into how the method could be applied to a growing list of issues and addictions, and together we explored and mapped out its evolution. I was more than happy to have the responsibility of continuing this vital mission placed on my shoulders by Allen himself. It's a responsibility I accepted with humility, and one I take extremely seriously.

WHAT ARE OUR CREDENTIALS?

We've been treating behavioral issues and addictions all over the world with phenomenal success over the past 35 years. Easyway's senior team and I were inspired to join Allen's quest for one simple reason: his method saved our lives. Like every Allen Carr's Easyway Therapist in the world, we were all drawn to get involved in Easyway as a result of being set free from our own behavioral issues and addictions.

Allen reveled in helping people deal with a whole variety of issues, and many of those who were lucky enough to be helped were so inspired and grateful to him, they contacted him to offer their help to drive the method forward. It proved to be a fertile field from which to recruit, and it was a pleasure to work with Allen in assembling the most remarkable senior therapist team to set about the task of applying the method to as many issues as possible.

The varied background of behavioral issues and/or drug-taking history of Allen's senior therapist team, far from deterring Allen from recruiting them, encouraged him to do so. If he was impressed by your drive, enthusiasm, ability, and accomplishments, he considered it a superb bonus if you had previously experienced the misery of other issues to which Easyway could be applied. He was acutely aware that it would be extremely difficult to apply his method to the full range of behavioral issues and addictions without the direct involvement of people who had used the method to set themselves free from them. Whether it be weight or eating issues, fear of flying, gambling, debt, heroin, cocaine, cannabis, alcohol or nicotine addiction, direct, up close, and personal experience of those issues enabled Allen and his team to develop the method accordingly.

This book is the direct result of our determination to apply Allen's brilliant method as far and as wide as possible, and I'm delighted that we have finally provided the solution for anyone whose life has been blighted by sleep issues. And we've done so with confidence. How can we do that?

SIMPLE: THIS METHOD WORKS!

Our motivation for putting the method down in writing was to enable anyone, anywhere in the world, regardless of their level of wealth, to benefit from *Allen Carr's Easy Way to Better Sleep*. This isn't simply a transcript of our successful Online Video Program for better sleep—that is a dynamic audiovisual presentation of the method by one of the most senior Allen Carr's Easyway Therapists in the world, and is supported by telephone and email support for the few who require it. But it is certainly the next best thing.

Make no mistake, this book is a complete program in itself.

I'm aware that many people who are unfamiliar with the method, or who have never met people who have benefited from Easyway, assume that some of the claims made about it are far-fetched or exaggerated. That was certainly my reaction when I first heard them. I was incredibly fortunate to have had my life saved by Allen Carr. There is no doubt that had I not come into contact with Allen and his amazing method in the late 1990s I wouldn't have made it to the 21st century—let alone be here today.

I'm incredibly proud to have headed up the team that, over the past 24 years, has taken Allen's method from Berlin to Bogotá, from New Zealand to New York, from Sydney to Santiago and beyond.

I still take pleasure in deflecting all the praise and acclaim straight back to the great man himself; it's all because of Allen Carr.

The method is as pure, as bright, as adaptable, and as effective as it's ever been, allowing us to apply it to a whole host of addictions and issues. Whether it's sleep, cannabis, cocaine, heroin, alcohol or sugar addiction, gambling, junk spending, fear of flying, mindfulness, or even digital / social-media addiction, the method guides those who need help in a simple, relatable, plain-speaking way.

Please don't mistake Allen Carr's Easyway method for some kind of "Jack of all trades." As you're about to discover for yourself, there is no doubt that it truly is the master of all behavioral issues and addictions.

Now, without further delay, let me pass you into the safest of hands—Allen Carr and his "Easyway."

Chapter 1

SICK AND TIRED

AN INSOMNIA EPIDEMIC •A MATTER OF URGENCY
•WHAT'S KEEPING YOU AWAKE? •A METHOD THAT WORKS

When did we lose the ability to sleep? When did it become such an effort?

Sleep is, or should be, the most natural thing in the world—as effortless as breathing. But the fact that you're reading this book suggests that sleep is not coming easily to you. Not at all. The hours of deep, refreshing sleep that we all need to function at our best are just not happening for you. Either you struggle to get to sleep or your sleep is disturbed—and it's having a huge impact on you.

You've tried everything, from vigorous exercise to soothing baths to herbal drinks to meditation, pills, patches, and potions, but the problem persists. It doesn't matter how tired you get, sleep eludes you. And when it doesn't—it's probably not quality sleep. In fact, the problem seems to get worse the more tired you become. It's as if you're held back by some monster that takes great delight in torturing you by depriving you of the rest you so badly crave.

It's not just a problem at night, either. Long-term sleep problems take their toll in the daytime too. You feel tired and find it hard to motivate yourself to carry out everyday tasks.

Your judgment suffers. You feel hunger more keenly and snack more, leading to weight gain, and you begin to lean heavily on stimulants in an attempt to keep you going. In extreme examples your relationships may suffer, your work suffers, and you struggle to maintain a social life.

Sleep deprivation creates a fear, too—not just the fears and stresses you experience as you lie awake at night fretting, but anxiety at the prospect of another sleepless night. That anxiety can dog you throughout the day, and it gets more intense with tiredness. It's a vicious circle. You can't sleep, you feel tired, you get anxious, your anxiety keeps you awake… and on it goes.

How can you break the cycle and get back to enjoying that gorgeous promise, that wonderful lure, of a good night's sleep?

AN INSOMNIA EPIDEMIC

Suffering from sleep deprivation is a lonely experience. Nobody can share it with you. You lie awake at night with your thoughts running around your brain, demanding attention: problems that need solutions; obligations that need to be fulfilled; relationships that need to be fixed; worries whirring around your mind like phantoms… Nobody can help shoulder the burden. It is a problem that leaves the sufferer feeling desperately isolated and helpless.

The paradox, though, is that millions of people are suffering just as you are. In fact, it would be hard to find anyone who has not experienced sleep deprivation and the anxieties described above at some time or other. We all know what it feels like and how it affects us. So why is it that for some of us these are brief periods in our lives, which we can pass through without too much trouble, but others get stuck, as if caught in a trap, which tightens the more we struggle?

Millions of people will recognize this description. Depending on which scientific study you read, chronic insomnia affects from 10 percent to 50 percent of the world's adult population. Even at the lower end, that's a lot of people struggling to do the thing that should come most naturally every night.

There are many theories as to why this should be. Some put it down to our obsessive use of electronic devices, messing with our minds and preventing us from being able to "switch off" at night. Some blame it on diet and the amount of unhealthy food and drinks we consume these days. Others align the insomnia epidemic with the prevalence of addiction—to everything from nicotine, alcohol, and other drugs to gambling, shopping, and playing video games. Others say it has to do with our stressful lifestyles and our inability to unwind.

None of these things help, so we will address them in this book and explain how you can give yourself a better chance of a good night's sleep by making some simple lifestyle and behavior changes. But none of them is solely to blame either.

Insomnia is not a new problem. It has been a common complaint since doctors' records began. We know that sleep disorders become more prevalent with age and certain diseases and physiological conditions, such as diabetes and menopause. It also affects both sexes, although women are about 40 percent more likely to experience it than men.

All this might seem very confusing. "What chance do I have of getting a good night's sleep if I'm living through an insomnia epidemic in which everything I do contributes to my inability to sleep?" But look at it another way. None of these studies claims that people like you are just doomed to suffer from sleep deprivation for the rest of their lives. That means there is a way out of the trap. You just need some help to find it.

A MATTER OF URGENCY

By picking up this book you have made an important move. You've taken a positive step to get help with your condition. I doubt that this book is your first port of call in that regard, and imagine that having made previous attempts to address it, perhaps even with some success before slipping back into the trap, you might be skeptical or might have even given up any hope at all of breaking free of this awful, debilitating suffering. Because sleep loss makes us tired, it takes away the energy we need to tackle our problems. Have you ever felt tired at the wheel of a car? It's terrifying how powerful the feeling can be. I'm not talking about feeling a little fatigued, but about having to battle to keep your eyes open. Part of your brain is telling you to stay alert, concentrate; you're in control of what is effectively a lethal weapon and you need to keep your wits about you. Another part is saying, "Close your eyes. Sleep. Let yourself go." If you're lucky, the "stay alert" part wins—but it can be a real struggle and, tragically, for too many people, the "sleep" part has the final say. You might have moments like that yourself, which seem to impose a special form of double torture;

there are times when you can barely stay awake but simply cannot allow yourself to sleep, and other moments when you're desperate for sleep but, no matter how tired you feel, you cannot achieve it.

When your problem is not driving a car but sleep deprivation itself, that's when you start to feel trapped. You know you need to do something about it, but you just don't have the energy for that now. That's why it's great news that you made the decision to read this book. It wasn't a hard step, but it will prove to be a vital one.

Because sleep loss is a serious threat to you and the world around you.

We've talked about the effects that sleep loss can have on you during the day, but being tired and irritable is just the tip of the iceberg. Suffering from insufficient sleep makes you more likely to wreck your car or have an accident at work or at home. In other words, it weaponizes you to cause havoc wherever you go.

The long-term threat to your health is another good reason for taking action now. Insufficient sleep increases your risk of cancer, obesity, diabetes, depression, and hypertension. This isn't just an inconvenience we're talking about—it's a life-threatening condition, and you've taken a huge step to address it now!

WHAT'S KEEPING YOU AWAKE?

Can you put your finger on the thing that is depriving you of sleep? Perhaps you find it hard to fall asleep at night. You can feel absolutely exhausted but still sleep doesn't come. For some reason the switch that turns the lights off in your mind just won't flip. You don't necessarily have to have a lot on your mind for this to happen. Your mind can feel bewilderingly blank, just waiting for sleep, but it doesn't come. And as we all know, sleep is not something you can force. You can't will yourself to sleep—that's like trying to pull on opposite ends of a rope at the same time.

Maybe you can get to sleep, but you wake up in the wee hours and can't drift off again. What is it that wakes you up? Is it a physical disturbance in the room that arouses you, and then the thoughts come streaming in? Perhaps the cat has a habit of jumping on you at 2 o'clock in the morning and then you're awake for the next two hours.

Or is it a thought that wakes you up? A nasty, pointy little anxiety that prods you awake in a panic and keeps your mind racing for hours. As you read through the book you will develop a better understanding of how sleep works, how the mind behaves before, during, and coming out of sleep, and how you can use this understanding to prepare yourself for a good night's rest.

What's addiction got to do with a sleep issue?
So how can you break the cycle and get back to that gorgeous promise of a good night's sleep? Moreover, how can a book help you break the cycle and sleep as nature intended?

This book takes an approach to tackling sleep deprivation that you haven't come across before—unless, that is, you have used Allen Carr's Easyway to quit smoking, drinking, gambling, overeating, or any of the other addictions and issues that this method has helped tens of millions of people overcome.

You might be wondering how the same method that helps people quit smoking can help with sleep deprivation. Notwithstanding the fact that smoking is a major cause of sleeping disorders—as are other drugs like caffeine and alcohol, as well as the consumption of refined sugar and processed carbohydrates—there is a big difference in the way the two conditions are perceived. We tend to blame smokers for their addiction to nicotine—they bring it on themselves; whereas sleep loss is something that just happens to you—it's bad luck. We tend to view smokers as perpetrators and insomniacs as victims.

This is not the case. The fact is that, in most cases, insomnia, like smoking, is brought on by any number of lifestyle and behavior choices. OK, some of those choices, such as working night shifts and traveling long-haul for work may seem less like free will than, say, smoking and drinking, but they are choices nonetheless. There are alternatives, and we need to apply our free will and logic to find them.

We will look at those choices in more detail. For now, it's important that you begin with the acceptance that you are not a victim. Put aside the idea that you are "an insomniac" and replace it with the fact that you currently "suffer from insomnia." Your condition is curable, and you have the power to free yourself.

Many people believe that addiction to nicotine and other drugs is a physical condition that needs a physical solution, such as nicotine patches/gum or e-cigarettes. In fact, addiction is 99 percent psychological. It controls the mind through a combination of brainwashing and the chemical effect of the drug. The way to cure it is by unraveling the brainwashing that convinces the addict that they enjoy the effects of the drug. In doing that, they discover the true nature of addiction: that it's based on the addict being fooled into believing that they get a genuine form of pleasure or benefit from taking the drug.

The physical withdrawal from nicotine is so slight as to be almost imperceptible. It is the effect the drug has on the brain, the addict's belief system, that gets them hooked. It's almost entirely psychological—behavioral rather than chemical.

The psychological influence on sleep is much more widely understood. If you can tackle the mental barriers to sleep, you will find a way to overcome your insomnia. That's how Easyway works. It helps you change your mindset, releasing you from the trap that keeps you awake at night.

A METHOD THAT WORKS

The good thing about sleep-loss sufferers versus addicts is that you are, as a general rule, open to trying new things. Nicotine and alcohol addicts are perhaps more stubborn, harder to convince that they even have a problem, let alone that their addiction can be overcome without having to rely on willpower or having to endure a painful, unpleasant transition period (known in addiction circles as "withdrawal"). To do that, it's essential that they understand how the minor chemical addiction combines with the larger psychological and behavioral aspects to keep them hooked.

One of my main revelations was that willpower, far from being the key to overcoming addiction and behavioral problems, actually makes them worse. You will learn why that is later in this book. For now, the good news is that you won't need willpower to make this method work, nor will you have to make any sacrifices or go through any miserable transition period. I would ask you to forgive any cross-references that I might make between sleep issues and addictions or other behavioral issues to which I have applied Easyway. I'll keep them to a minimum and will only mention them when they help explain or illustrate an important point. I promise you that they will be relevant to your condition.

Other than that, all you have to do is read this book from start to finish and follow all the instructions.

As you progress through the book, you will find a series of instructions. It's essential that you follow them. The instructions are fundamental to Easyway and they work like the combination of a safe. Unlocking a safe is easy if you know the right combination of numbers. Miss any one of them, though, or apply them in the wrong order, and the door will not spring open.

That's all you have to do with this method. Follow it in order and in its entirety. It's that easy. And it works. Allen Carr's Easyway has helped tens of millions of people quit smoking, drinking, gambling, overeating, and a host of other conditions where traditional methods have failed. It has rescued countless addicts from despair, when so-called experts had told them they lacked the willpower or that they just had an addictive personality.

We have enjoyed phenomenal success with this method around the world for one simple reason:

IT WORKS!

And so to your first instruction:

You must follow ALL the instructions. In order.

You know why. The combination lock will not open if you miss a number, use a number out of sequence, or skip straight to the end in search of the key. The whole book is the key and must be used as designed.

The second instruction is:

Keep an open frame of mind.

It was an open mind that enabled you to pick up this book in the first place. Keep believing. Put aside any thought that you are "an insomniac," doomed to suffer sleep deprivation for the rest of your life. You were not born with insomnia. You were not predestined to suffer sleep loss. You suffer it for a reason, or a variety of reasons, and you can undo the influence of those reasons and walk out of the trap just as easily as you fell into it.

This book will help you achieve the mindset necessary to restore your sleep balance and feel the benefit in all aspects of your life, without willpower or a miserable or demanding transition period. As you read through the book and your belief in your ability to conquer your sleep problem increases, you will feel a growing sense of joy, optimism, and energy.

Embrace it! This is the way we are meant to feel.

Chapter 2

THE SLEEP INSTINCT

WHAT HAPPENS WHEN WE SLEEP

It seems like a silly question, but have you ever wondered why we sleep? Why is sleep so important? What happens to us during those resting hours? And what are the consequences of failing to get a good night's sleep?

Until fairly recently, we believed sleep was the brain shutting down to rest and recuperate at the end of the day. Now we know that the brain doesn't shut down during sleep; in fact, it becomes remarkably active, with different neurons acting to trigger physical and mental recovery.

We all know that blissful feeling of drowsiness. Scientists chalk this up to a chemical called adenosine, which builds up while we are awake and breaks down while we sleep. If you take naps during the day, you dispel some of your adenosine, which could make it harder to get to sleep at night.

The "sleep hormone" melatonin is a chemical released by a gland in the brain called the pineal gland. Its production is responsive to light, so it is triggered as it gets dark and stops being released as it gets light again. This clever natural process is what controls our sleep rhythms, in tune with night and day.

There are two basic types of sleep: rapid eye movement (REM) sleep and non-REM sleep. When we fall asleep, we go into the first stages of non-REM sleep, known as light sleep.

After about 30 minutes, we fall into stage 3 non-REM sleep, a deeper sleep state, during which the body starts its restoration process. There are four stages of non-REM sleep in all, the fourth being an even deeper sleep state than stage 3.

It is during these deep sleep stages that the body synthesizes protein to build cells and make us stronger. In children and young people, this is when growth takes place. This sleep is also good for your cardiovascular system. Heart rate falls and blood pressure drops.

SLEEP FACT

Sleep has a direct effect on heart health. In the spring, when the clocks go forward and we lose an hour of sleep, the number of heart attacks shoots up by 24 percent the next day. In the fall, when we gain an hour, they decrease by 21 percent. A similar effect is seen with road accidents, suicides, and even the severity of criminal sentences. It all points to the vital benefits of sleep.

Studies of brain activity during non-REM sleep have suggested that, during these deep sleep states, you replay the day's experiences like a projector running at 20 times the normal speed, saving them in your memory bank as you go along.

Between these deep sleep stages, we come up into a short period of REM sleep, also known as dream sleep. During REM sleep, you rebuild your immune system and your brain activates an extraordinary process of thought analysis, which we know as dreams.

This apparently chaotic mental process is believed to be the brain analyzing the experiences of the day and looking for connections with past experiences already stored in the memory bank. During deep sleep, you take the information you have learned and you save it. This is why dreams can be so random and full of strange connections. It is also why we can sometimes come up with answers to previously baffling problems while we are asleep.

The brain is very active during REM sleep—more active in parts than when you're awake, in fact—and if you acted out some of your thoughts, you could end up in some very strange and possibly dangerous situations. To prevent this, the brain cleverly switches off all motor signals to the body, effectively paralyzing you during REM sleep.

So we sleep in order to restore, rebuild, memorize, and analyze. To illustrate how important these processes are, let's look at what happens when we're deprived of a good night's sleep.

THE BENEFITS OF SLEEP

During deep non-REM sleep we replay the lessons of the day and consign them to memory. That's why a good night's sleep is important not only for adults but also essential for children and students to learn and retain knowledge.

But sleep also plays an important part in preparing the brain for learning. Studies have shown that sleep deprivation attacks a part of the brain called the hippocampus—the part that controls memory—causing a 40 percent reduction in the ability of the brain to make new memories.

Memory loss is a symptom of aging, as is sleep loss. Coincidence? Absolutely not. Poor sleep is now known to contribute not just to the scatterbrained loss of memory that we associate with getting older, but also to the more severe conditions of Alzheimer's disease and dementia.

The glymphatic system is a recently discovered feature of our biology, designed for cleansing toxins from the central nervous system. It is activated during sleep by powerful bursts of electrical activity in the brain, protecting and refreshing your capacity for learning and memory every day.

When the glymphatic system is not fully activated, toxins build up. There is strong evidence linking this with the development of Alzheimer's disease in later life. Similarly, a lack of REM sleep, or disturbed REM sleep, has been shown to increase the risk of developing Parkinson's disease.

Even people who don't have a sleep issue greatly underestimate the importance of sleep, and have no idea that they are, in fact, damaging the length, quality, and enjoyment of their future lives by routinely depriving themselves of adequate sleep. A huge number of people do not get a minimum of eight hours of sleep in their schedule, not realizing the harm they're doing to themselves. It's not that they can't sleep for longer but, through ignorance, they simply choose not to! At least you are aware of your sleep issue and the beautiful truth that the key to your release is in your hands.

These facts can be frightening for anyone who is suffering from sleep disruption, but on the positive side, it's wonderful to know that you have the situation in hand and that not only will you be releasing yourself from the nightmare of poor sleep and the tiredness, irritability, work, and relationship issues it causes, but you'll also have some even more wonderful health bonuses to enjoy for the rest of your life. Sleep disorders can be taken as indicators of critical health conditions later in life, as much as 20 years down the road, giving us the opportunity to take preventative action. In other words, sleep serves as a warning mechanism.

Alertness

When you get a good night's sleep, you are less prone to tiredness during the day. That might sound obvious, and not a big deal—we can all deal with feeling a little tired, can't we?

Up to a point. Whether you take care of children all day or deal with the fine margins between success and failure in your workplace, whether your walk to work or take public transportation, lack of sleep impairs your judgment, safety, and wellbeing. Tiredness takes on a whole new level of danger when you operate machinery at work or get behind the wheel of a car.

The law is very strict on the consumption of alcohol and other drugs when driving, but tiredness causes more deaths on the road than alcohol or drugs. Drunk driving is highly dangerous because it slows down your reaction time. In fact, driving when tired is proven to be comparable to drunk driving. But when you fall asleep at the wheel, you don't react at all.

Being distracted by fatigue or even drifting off for just two seconds can be enough to swerve into the path of oncoming traffic. Alcohol may cause more accidents than sleeping or tiredness at the wheel but, tragically, accidents tend to be more deadly with the latter.

Emotional health

It's common knowledge that sleep deprivation makes us irritable and moody, but that's just the tip of a horrifically tragic iceberg. At the other extreme is an increase in depression, anxiety, and suicide.

Deep in the center of the brain are two almond-shaped regions called the amygdala (from the Greek for almond). Their job is to regulate our emotions, build emotional connections with our memories, and help with decision-making and reward processing.

Scientists monitoring the reactivity of the amygdala have found a disturbing 60 percent increase resulting from sleep deprivation. At the same time, the prefrontal cortex, which keeps the emotional brain in check, becomes deactivated by lack of sleep.

As a result of this hyperactivity in the amygdala and lack of restraining influence from the prefrontal cortex, our behavior can become unstable and irrational. We can sway from grumpy to hysterical, become more demanding and unreasonable.

In normal circumstances we shrug it off as just being tired and irritable, but these responses are similar to brain behavior observed in severe psychiatric disorders. Sleep deprivation is not just a symptom of these disorders, but an important predictor too, sounding the alarm for conditions that could develop into depression, Post Traumatic Stress Disorder (PTSD) and suicide if they remain unchecked.

You don't need to be worried about this information. Doing so won't help resolve your sleep issues; in fact, it would make them worse. Instead, release from these considerations and risks becomes a huge bonus to enjoy when you are free.

Immunity

Sleep and the immune system have a bidirectional relationship. In other words, sleep affects the immune system, and the immune system affects sleep.

There are two types of immunity: that which you're born with and that which you adopt. It's important for both to be in balance.

During sleep, the immune system is strengthened and becomes more active. The natural killer cells, which identify pathogens and destroy them, need sleep to increase in number. In fact, just one night of poor sleep can reduce immune cell activity by 70 percent.

So when we have a bad night's sleep, we don't just become irritable, we become more vulnerable to illness too. This goes far beyond just feeling run down. There is a strong connection between sleep deprivation and numerous forms of cancer, so much so that the World Health Organization, whom we work with, has classified shift work as a probable carcinogen! That's not to say you should consider leaving your job if you enjoy, or are restricted to, shift work. It's just important to emphasize the absolute requirement for as much focus to be directed toward obtaining healthy levels of sleep as you might place on diet and exercise.

It's extraordinary to think that people deprive themselves of adequate sleep in order to get a session in at the gym before going to work. In health terms, it's like attempting to fill a leaky bucket with water. Going to the gym is a great thing to do—but fitting it in around healthy sleep is essential.

Attractiveness

You're familiar with the expression "beauty sleep." Well, it's true. Sleep really does make you more attractive.

It's no revelation that sleep, or lack of it, affects the way you look in the morning. Dark bags under the eyes, pallid skin, lank hair, a general lack of vibrancy—we can all spot someone who's had a bad night's sleep.

But is that necessarily less beautiful? Well, yes, as it turns out. Researchers in Sweden took photographs of individuals after a good night's sleep and after a bad night's sleep, then showed them to a panel of judges, who had no idea what the experiment was about. They consistently rated the sleep-deprived versions as less attractive. Ouch!

DO ANIMALS SUFFER FROM INSOMNIA?

All animals sleep. Some, like dolphins, sleep with one half of their brain at a time, so the other half can stay alert for predators and other survival needs. Others, like the bullfrog, sleep annually during hibernation. For all animals, sleep is the mechanism for resetting brain and body health.

Not all animals need eight to nine hours of quality sleep a night, as humans do, but they all get what they need. All except us humans. We are the only species that suffers from chronic insomnia or that routinely, voluntarily overrides its minimum requirement for sleep. To be clear—with regard to the latter, I'm not focusing on the occasional late night. We all have those. I'm focusing on the huge number of people who resist adequate sleep every single night.

As with obesity and addiction, those other blights of modern living, sleep disorder is a uniquely human condition brought on by uniquely human behaviors. We are the only species that fights the instinct to sleep and the only species that deliberately interrupts our own sleep in the morning, bringing it to an unnatural end with an alarm.

The way we sleep is far from the way that nature intended. We have talked about melatonin. This hormone reacts to the light, inducing sleep when the sun goes down and waking us when it rises. But who goes to bed and rises with the sun these days?

We have chosen to ignore the natural signals for sleeping and we wonder why we suffer from insomnia and poor health.

Don't worry, this isn't leading up to an instruction to sleep when the sun goes down and wake when it rises. But this point alone illustrates how our lifestyle choices create unnatural conditions for a good night's sleep. In order to cure your insomnia, you need to do what you can to keep those sleep-disruptive lifestyle choices to a minimum.

Going to sleep with the sun is impractical with our modern working timetable, but there are plenty of other choices you can change without putting your livelihood at risk. In fact, most of them will leave you better off—physically, mentally, and financially.

MOTHER NATURE'S GUIDE

When you start to learn about how sleep works and the functions performed during sleep, you have to admit that the human being is an incredible machine. It is infinitely more complex than a car, a plane, or even the most complex, advanced fighter jet. And yet there is a flaw—a flaw that causes all those miserable human-made problems like addiction, obesity, and insomnia.

The essential difference between humans and other animals, all of which sleep soundly at the exact point of night, or day, that is appropriate for them, is that their behavior is dominated by instinct. We have instincts too, but we also have the added faculty of intelligence. We can remember past experiences and apply the knowledge gained from them to new situations. We also have the ability to communicate this knowledge and hand it down to future generations.

It is this facility to learn and develop by a process of deduction that has put us way ahead of the rest of the animal kingdom. But this superiority has also given us the belief that we are in control of our own destiny. When our instinct and our intellect are at odds, we tend to put our faith in intellect. This is the flaw in the human machine.

Instinct is an unconscious response and, as such, it is something we don't really understand or trust. When our instinct and intellect are in conflict, we find it easier to make a reasoned argument in support of the intelligent course of action, even when there is overwhelming evidence that this is the wrong option.

Let's take an example: say you have to stake your professional reputation on the outcome of a football game. You can seek the advice of two people. One of them is the most intelligent person on the planet, who has predicted the results of 100 games and achieved a 75 percent success rate; the other is by all appearances an unsophisticated, unscholarly, incoherent misfit who has made a million predictions and gotten them all correct. Whom would you trust?

Because we don't understand our instincts, we regard them as hit or miss—a hunch perhaps, or an old wives' tale. But instinct is not hit or miss, it is the result of three million years of trial and error. It is what enables other animals to breed and to feed without harm. Wild animals don't have eating disorders like humans.

They don't get obese. They don't consume poisons. Instinct is their guide.

We talk about the miracle of childbirth. The reason it appears to be a miracle is because the reproduction of life is way beyond the capacity of our intelligence. The fact is that the achievements of the human race, no matter how great, pale into insignificance next to the achievements of Mother Nature.

With any machine, if you want to know how it works, the best person to ask is the person who designed it. The same goes for the human body. If you want to understand how it is designed to work—or, more to the point, why it appears not to be working, there is no higher authority than Mother Nature's guide.

In other words, listen to your instincts!

You're now ready for the third instruction:

If someone gives you advice that contradicts the clear intentions of Mother Nature, regardless of how eminent or qualified that person may be, IGNORE IT!

I call this instruction "the Monkey Wrench." Regardless of how highly you regard another person's expertise, taking their advice over what you instinctively feel is as misguided as hiring a monkey rather than a mechanic to fix your car.

Intellect isn't the only thing that sets us apart from the rest of the animal kingdom. We are also the only species on the planet that has sleep problems; 99.999 percent of all the creatures on Earth get all the sleep they need, whenever they need it. Obviously, it can't be that complicated—and yet the most intelligent species on the planet is struggling to figure it out.

If you're dismissing what I say about instinct when comparing humans to animals, be aware that the only animals that suffer from sleep issues or weight issues are those that rely on humans for their food, environment, and care (pets), or those that feed on our refined sugar/processed carb-laden food waste (pigeons and vermin, etc).

Is it possible that, by some ironic twist, intelligence has become the very reason for our ignorance? Could the fact that we are so much more intelligent than any other species have led us away from the truth? Have we observed the animal kingdom and decided that we know better?

Why is it that we look to nutritionists, for example, to tell us what to eat to keep in shape? Animals don't need nutritionists— they know instinctively what they should and shouldn't eat. And so did we, once upon a time.

The aim of this book is to make sleep simple. Right now you're probably thinking that, if it were simple, you would have fixed it by now. When is anything in life ever that simple? I refer you to 99.999 percent of the animal kingdom, which finds it simple to get the sleep they need.

The undeniable fact is that, from a fairly young age, we fight sleep. We will look at the reasons why in the next chapter. Before we do, it is important to deal with two possible misconceptions about the Easyway method.

1. It isn't magic. Many people who have quit smoking, vaping, cocaine addiction and the like with this method

describe it as such, but that is purely a figure of speech. There is nothing complex or mysterious about Easyway; it is plain common sense.

2. It doesn't involve any mind games or illusions. On the contrary, it works by dispelling illusions. There are no mind games involved—just plain, simple logic. Once you see it, nothing will be able to change your mind.

Chapter 3

THE FIGHT AGAINST SLEEP

•LATE NIGHTS •THE WORK ETHIC •WHAT'S YOUR DEVICE? •STRESS •ANXIETY •DIET •STIMULANTS •CHOICE

Sleep is essential for us to restore our immunity, rebuild our strength, retain what we have learned and analyze information. It is as crucial as eating, keeping active, and protecting our mental health. And yet, just like those vital aspects of life, our intellect has led us to believe that we can go without sleep.

LATE NIGHTS

As infants we sleep exactly when, and for as long as, we need to. We might not sleep through the night because there are other demands, like hunger or physical security, that wake us, but it's very hard to deprive a baby of sleep.

It's not long, however, before the urge to fight sleep kicks in. As children, we get excited by the idea of staying up late. Being allowed to stay up past our bedtime is regarded as a special treat. Why? When a child goes to bed late, they upset their natural rhythm, their sleep is disrupted, and they suffer.

Would you give your child a cigarette as a treat? There is really no difference. We have established that disrupted sleep leads to serious medical problems later in life. The kindest thing any parent can do for their child is to protect them from these threats by helping them get a good night's sleep EVERY NIGHT.

In our teens, late nights take on an even more compelling status. They become a badge of honor. Who can pull an all-nighter? As if missing a whole night's sleep is somehow clever or tough! What's clever or tough about denying your body and mind the chance to restore and rebuild? It's the most ridiculous, debilitating, self-inflicted punishment imaginable! We've all done it.

Maybe that's the appeal. We do become masochistic in our adolescent years. Alcohol, cigarettes, and other drugs are all poisons that we choose to try, thinking we're being grown-up and free, when actually we're walking into a trap that enslaves us to addiction, sleep disorders, and other miserable conditions, often for the rest of our lives.

I'm not suggesting that, in an ideal world, young people should live like monks. It's just important to see how we've grown to consider sleep so unimportant, how we've neglected it, and how we go about solving our sleep issues the wrong way.

THE WORK ETHIC

We live in an incredible age of technological convenience and labor-saving devices. We look back at history and consider ourselves lucky that we weren't living in an era when everything was done by hand, people suffered from dreadful diseases, and life was generally harder. We think we have progressed. We think we have a better standard of living. We are kidding ourselves!

The average adult works longer hours today than they did 100 years ago. Despite all the conveniences and labor-saving devices, it seems we are compelled to work more than the next person, to get ahead or to avoid the stigma of laziness.

In 1910, the average American adult enjoyed 8.25 hours sleep a night. Today that number is closer to 6.75 hours. And the impact on our health and wellness is stark. Dementia, Alzheimer's, Parkinson's, cancer, heart disease, diabetes… future generations will look back and pity us for our hardship and the terrible diseases we suffered.

Or perhaps they will continue the downward spiral, deluding themselves that they are making progress.

It's not just adults who are working longer and losing sleep either. Starting at the age of five, children are now getting two hours' less sleep per night than they did 100 years ago. Two hours! That's nearly a quarter of the sleep a child needs to be healthy. If you took away a quarter of the food a child needs simply to remain healthy, it would be rightly branded as cruelty. In fact, modern living has caused more than one generation of children to be brought up on artificial additives, flavorings, refined sugar and processed carbohydrates: junk masquerading as food. Their malnourishment, of which the obesity epidemic is a symptom, is another issue entirely… until it comes to addressing the sleep issues they experience.

It is perfectly natural for children to want to stay up late. It is part of the process of cutting the apron strings and establishing their independence. They want to go to bed later and wake up later. The trouble is, they are allowed the first part but not the second. There is no time to make up for it in the morning.

Research has shown that a child's brain doesn't start functioning fully until 10am, but school starts an hour or two earlier than that! We are pushing our children to be more and more academic while disabling the number one tool they need to learn!

We regard it as a function of our civilized society that we no longer get up for work with the sun, as our ancestors did.

Instead, we have decided that it is best to be the only species on earth that interrupts its sleep with an alarm, so we can get to work at the same time, every working day of the year.

There are tribes on Earth that do still live by the sun. They find it baffling that anyone should interrupt their night's sleep before it is complete. And guess what: only 1 or 2 percent of them suffer from insomnia, compared to as much as 30 percent in the so-called "developed" world.

Again, it is our intellect that has brought this about. We plan work and school timetables according to what we think we need to get done, never according to our natural rhythms, the rising and setting of the sun or the basic need for a full night's sleep. As work builds up, as it always does, sleep is the first thing that suffers.

WHAT'S YOUR DEVICE?

The digital revolution has changed our lives in many wonderful ways. During the COVID-19 pandemic, for example, the ability to communicate from home was a life-saver—literally, in some cases.

It enabled us to isolate but still keep in contact with others. It played a key part in allowing the world to keep working, families and loved ones to stay in touch, children to keep learning, and the wheels of commerce to keep turning.

But digital devices have been disastrous for our sleep. We just don't seem able to put them down.

Digital devices and their apps have been designed to be as addictive as any drug, and we have a growing number of people contacting our seminar centers seeking help for digital addiction. The biggest concern seems to be fear of missing out (FOMO), a natural human trait that has been exploited by social media to keep us hooked day and night.

Why is this a problem? There are two main reasons that we know of. The first is the blue light that is emitted from the screens of smartphones, tablets etc. This blue light delays the release of melatonin, the hormone that triggers our sleep reflex. In other words, screen use keeps you awake at night when you would naturally be feeling sleepy.

Blue light also disrupts your REM sleep—the dream sleep state—in which we process thoughts and information and cleanse the toxins from the brain. In other words, blue light is a threat to long-term mental health.

The second reason is that our obsessive use of smart devices causes anxiety. The fact that we check our phones so often is driven by the anxiety of missing out on something we deem to be important. A business memo… A message from a friend… A joke that's doing the rounds… A piece of news…

Furthermore, if you keep your phone or tablet by the bed, you suffer from what is called "anticipatory anxiety" the moment you wake up—the anticipation of checking your device to see what's going on. As soon as your phone lights up, a barrage of information floods in and your brain is hit with the challenge of taking it all in. Or deciding what to take in and what to ignore.

This is hugely stressful and counterproductive to a peaceful night's sleep.

Speaking of which…

STRESS

Like working late and depriving yourself of sleep, stress is often confused as something to admire. "Wow! That must be stressful for her," is a subtext for, "Wow! She must be important." Somehow we have adopted the notion that stress is a sign of being smart, important, hardworking, influential. Sure, a lot of jobs that fit that description are stressful, but the problem is that we assume the inverse to be true too. If you're not stressed, you can't be smart, important, hardworking, or influential. Of course, this is nonsense.

After all, we spend half our time trying to de-stress. We try yoga, meditation, fitness, sports, dancing, music… all kinds of things to soothe this terrible thing called stress. We really ought to make up our minds: is stress a good thing or a bad thing?

In fact, both are true. Stress is one of the clever functions of the incredible human machine. It is an instinctive survival mechanism, which is triggered when we are in danger. Stress causes the release of hormones to raise the heart rate and pump more blood to the muscles, so we are ready to run or fight if necessary. Without stress, we would have been easy meat for the saber-toothed tiger and some other species would now be the dominant creature on Earth.

Stress becomes a bad thing when it is triggered by fears that are not a threat to our survival. Work pressure, relationship problems, stage fright… you could name any number of stressful situations. They happen on a daily basis. We don't tackle these problems as we would a saber-toothed tiger—through fight or flight—but our central nervous system nevertheless responds in the same way, raising those hormone levels.

This is OK if it happens from time to time, but because we put ourselves through these stressful situations day after day, the effect on sleep is devastating. An ongoing state of stress-hormone arousal can delay the onset of sleep and bring on anxiety at night, which also keeps us awake. The loss of sleep adds a further layer of stress and it becomes a vicious circle. The only way to break it is to, as much as possible, limit or avoid stressful situations for a while. It's certainly not useful to voluntarily maintain constant levels of stress as a result of our overuse, and inappropriate use, of technology—digital junk.

ANXIETY

Closely related to stress is anxiety. Stress is best defined as a physical response to external threats, whereas anxiety is the mental state that can arise from stress, or from purely psychological worries.

We can become anxious about real problems, such as having enough money to buy food and shelter, or about imaginary ones, like thinking our friends don't like us, or that our boss thinks we're incompetent, even though there is no evidence to back this up.

Anxiety is another clever function of the human machine. Our ancestors didn't just react when they heard the saber-toothed tiger roar; they knew when they were entering the tiger's domain and they would have been on high alert. That fear of something that *could* happen gave them a significant advantage, but today it means we lie awake fretting about matters that are neither life-threatening nor even, in some cases, real.

Anxiety and stress are not, in themselves, bad. We need them to survive. It's the causes of anxiety and stress that are becoming increasingly harmful: man-made causes like work, social acceptance, health and fitness, poor diet, behavioral issues, and addictions.

DIET

One of the ways we look to relieve stress and anxiety is through eating. "Comfort eating," we call it. And it's another vicious circle.

The foods we should be eating—the foods designed for us by Mother Nature—are fruit, vegetables, nuts, and seeds. These foods taste the best to us (think about all the artificial foods we make palatable by giving them a fruit flavor, or the processed carbohydrates (or meat for that matter) that we cover with vegetable- and herb-based sauces). Unlike refined sugar, processed or starchy carbohydrates, fresh fruit, fresh vegetables, nuts, and seeds are the easiest to digest. And guess what: they also happen to be the most nutritious.

But do we "comfort eat" fruit and nuts? Oh no! Cakes, ice cream, cookies, chocolate, potato chips, burgers, French fries, fried chicken, hot dogs, desserts... you'll find none of these foods in Mother Nature's guide, but we consume them in enormous quantities.

Why do we like them so much if they're so bad for us? Firstly, they manipulate our blood sugar levels which causes all kinds of problems and also because they are pumped full of sugar and salt, which are addictive, we get hooked on them. And whose idea was that? Human beings—in the pursuit of control and profit over other human beings.

If you think that sounds like a crackpot conspiracy theory, isn't that really the basis for the way we all live? Let's not be naïve. If you ran a company that sold food which contained next to zero nutritional value, wouldn't you make sure you put something in it to make it appear to taste good? If you still have your doubts, just look at the ingredients of any piece of junk food and ask yourself why the levels of sugar or salt (or both) are so high. It's to mask the otherwise bland nature of what we're being fed, and keep us coming back for more, with the food industry knowingly manipulating the addictive nature of refined sugar, and starchy and processed carbs; the last two also providing "bulk" in the products.

The evidence of our poor diet is clear to see in the ballooning level of diet-related conditions like obesity, diabetes, hypertension, and heart disease. Increasingly, studies into the relationship between diet and sleep are finding not only that a poor diet has a detrimental effect on sleep, but also that poor sleep has a detrimental effect on diet.

For example, high consumption of those unhealthy carbohydrates has been shown to increase the number of times we wake up at night and reduce the amount of deep sleep we get. On the other side of the circle, sleep deprivation causes us to eat more, and to eat higher-calorie foods, all without increasing the amount of exercise we do to burn it off.

STIMULANTS

A stimulant, as the name suggests, is any substance that stimulates the central nervous system, making you more alert and less inclined to sleep. Different stimulants do this in different ways. Caffeine, for example, prevents the buildup of adenosine, the chemical that makes us feel sleepy. Alcohol is normally a sedative, actually an anesthetic, which we go out of our way to often mix with sugary mixers or other ingredients, creating a weird contradiction in effect.

Alcohol's anesthetic "qualities" can produce drowsiness, but it is not the same as actual sleep. You lose consciousness, but your sleep is fragmented and your REM sleep is diminished. That's why you never wake up after a night of drinking alcohol feeling rested and refreshed.

Humans consume stimulants on a massive scale. And each time we do, we reduce our chances of getting a good night's sleep.

You don't need scientific evidence to support this statement. Most people have felt the disruptive effects of alcohol and caffeine on their sleep. But do you know just how disruptive these stimulants can be?

Take caffeine, the world's most universally popular stimulant. Caffeine has a half-life of around five hours, which means that five hours after drinking a cup, you still have the caffeine from half a cup of coffee in your system. After 10 hours, you still have a quarter of a cup.

So if you drink a cup of coffee a 2pm, you'll still be feeling the effects of a quarter of a cup at midnight. It's widely known that drinking any coffee at midnight is not going to help you get to sleep, but this shows a much more alarming fact. If you want to go to bed at 10pm and get a good night's sleep, it's best not to drink coffee after breakfast.

Even if you don't actually feel the effects of the caffeine at midnight, it will reduce the amount of deep sleep you get, making you feel tired in the morning. And what do you do to wake yourself up in the morning? Drink a cup of strong coffee!

One of the main reasons why we take so many stimulants is to counteract tiredness from a lack of sleep. Another vicious circle. Whether it's coffee, tea, chocolate, cookies, energy drinks, soda, alcohol, tobacco, energy supplements or illegal drugs, whatever temporary boost we get is inevitably followed by a crash. These extremes impact the brain's receptors and disrupt the natural process of sleep. That's why the more we rely on stimulants like caffeine, the less impact they have on the problem we're attempting to solve. Have you noticed how most heavy caffeine users always look exhausted? They think they're drinking coffee to get rid of the exhaustion they feel—they don't seem to realize that it's the daily bombardment of coffee that's made them feel that way. It's like trying to extinguish a flame with gasoline.

Often we consume stimulants without even knowing it. Refined salt and sugar are added to food and drinks, and there are other less familiar substances like guarana, taurine, and carnitine that have a similar effect. Our addiction to stimulants is a major reason for the insomnia epidemic.

CHOICE

In the next chapter we will look more closely at the vicious circle of fatigue and insomnia and how we become trapped in a cycle of sleep deprivation. The purpose of this chapter is to show that it is largely the choices we make in life—what we eat and drink, when we go to bed, when we wake up, how we connect with the world, our attitude to work—that give us sleep problems.

We are not born programmed to suffer from sleep deprivation. On the contrary, we are programmed to sleep just as naturally as we breathe. But human intellect presents us with this array of choices that all disrupt sleep, and our intellect tells us it's OK to go on choosing them.

Isn't it clear that in order to stand any chance of getting a good night's sleep, these choices have to change?

Simple? On paper, perhaps. But in reality? In your position? If it were simple, you would have done it by now, right?

So why do we find it so hard to quit the behaviors that cause us harm and revert to the lifestyle that nature designed for us? Why does that seem so far-fetched? Because just as sleep disruption feels like a trap, poor work-life balance, diet, addiction to stimulants, and digital devices are all forms of the same trap.

In order to break free you need to be aware of the trap and understand how it works.

Chapter 4

THE TRAP

TWO MONSTERS

Insomniacs often describe their struggle to sleep as like being caught in a trap, which tightens on them the more they struggle. The greater the need and desire for sleep, the greater the difficulty in achieving it.

Escaping from this trap would be simple if it were just a case of getting some physical rest. You could take a sedative, give your body a chance to recover and start again from scratch.

But there are two sides to the problem of sleep deficit: a physical side and a mental side. And the mental side is where the trap really comes into effect.

We all know the physical feeling of fatigue. We slow down, our muscles become restless, we yawn, our eyelids droop, we slouch, our shoulders drop, and we become clumsy. These are all symptoms of our central nervous system sending messages to the brain that it needs to sleep.

It's how the brain responds to these messages that is the key to whether we get the sleep we need. The natural response is to lie down and close our eyes. But is that what we do when we feel tired? Or do we look at the clock, and if it's not "bedtime," we watch another TV show or play another game and reach for something we believe is an effective stimulant to perk us up—a cup of coffee, an energy drink, a cigarette...

For a while those sleep messages are silenced, but as the stimulant wears off, they come flooding back louder than before. "I NEED SLEEP."

The physical sensation of fatigue can feel like a little monster, nagging away when you're trying to concentrate or relax and enjoy yourself. But the mental response is a big monster, which becomes impatient, irritable and, worst of all, irrational as the sleep messages come in.

It's the Big Monster that makes irrational choices, like having a cup of coffee when what you really need is sleep. It's the Big Monster that tells a teenager that studying all night is a great way to prepare for an exam. It's the Big Monster that tells us if we wake up earlier and go to bed later, we'll get more work done and alleviate our stress. And it's the Big Monster that keeps us awake at night, trying to solve problems when we're in the worst possible condition to do so.

The purpose of this book is to help you slay the Big Monster. The good news is, it's easy if you follow all the instructions. You don't need willpower. In fact, that's the last thing you need. All you need to do is reconnect with the natural instincts that enable all other animals to get the sleep they need night after night after night... or in the case of nocturnal beasts, day after day after day.

VICIOUS CIRCLES

In the last chapter we identified a number of vicious circles that disrupt sleep. There's the cycle we just mentioned, whereby we respond to fatigue by taking stimulants. This is such a common practice among human beings, it's a wonder anyone gets a decent night's sleep.

Stimulants disrupt sleep in two ways: first, they prevent us from getting sleep when we need it by counteracting our natural sleep hormones; and second, the energy spikes and crashes caused by stimulants corrupt the receptors in the brain, making them less effective at bringing on sleep when required.

Then there are the cycles between fatigue and anxiety and fatigue and stress. Anxiety and stress tend to go hand in hand, and they have many causes: work, money, time, relationships, obligations, disputes, responsibilities, ambitions, fears.... If you trigger your fight-or-flight response too often, you will become worn out, and that is exactly what happens with all the genuine stresses and anxieties we endure on a daily basis... not to mention the relentless wildness our bodies and brains endure when they are subjected to endless "shoot 'em up" games and the like on gaming platforms. It's repeated, endurance-level overstimulation on a massive scale. The same goes for our penchant for constant communication and social media. Long gone are the days when our relaxation in the evenings might be disturbed by the occasional phone call once or twice a week—now it's constant connectivity with, in many cases, people we don't even know!

Being worn out by stress and anxiety isn't a recipe for sleep.

On the contrary, raised levels of stress hormones counteract sleep. And to round the circle, knowing we're missing out on the sleep we need makes us stressed and anxious. Insomnia itself becomes a cause of anxiety.

Fatigue and diet are another vicious circle. The more tired we feel, the more junk we tend to eat. The more junk we eat, the less energy we have. The less energy we have, the more tired we feel.

Eating junk isn't just a consequence of feeling too tired to cook. Junk food (which really means any food that is not high in the nutrients we need) acts like a stimulant. We eat it in search of mental comfort as much as the need to satisfy hunger. It gives us an energy spike and then a crash, which is disastrous for our natural sleep functions and blood-sugar levels.

The increased use of tech devices is another vicious circle. Binge-watching TV, playing a never-ending video game, permanently plugged into social media… these all seem like easy leisure activities—the ideal kind of thing for winding down. So we turn more and more to our devices as fatigue sets in. It seems easier than reading a book or just lying there letting our thoughts wind down.

But we know that using devices has an intensely agitating effect on the brain, which is detrimental to sleep. So the devices we use to wind down when we're tired actually make us more tired and more inclined to reach for those devices and, with the fatigue it exacerbates, for those inefficient stimulants too.

These vicious circles are all consequences of the same mental trap. They create the feeling of being enslaved and helpless. But they are not traps that we are forced into at gunpoint. They are all created by bad lifestyle choices—which leads to the obvious question:

WHY DO WE MAKE SUCH TERRIBLE CHOICES?

Think about the influences in your life. Parents, family, teachers, friends, celebs, coworkers… Why do we follow these influences? It all starts at birth.

We are born vulnerable. We come into the world with a void that needs to be filled with security and love. As babies, we rely wholly on our parents to fill that void. In simple terms, they keep us alive and healthy. We couldn't do that for ourselves, so we trust our parents and the choices they make. But as we grow up, we begin to realize that our parents don't know everything, and they don't always tell the truth, either.

Now other influences play a part. Teachers start telling us things we didn't know, and we start to value their influence above that of our parents. Then we discover that teachers are not always right either. We look to our friends and copy what they do. And we look to celebrities: movie stars, rock stars, professional athletes— all those famous people who seem to have life under control and are doing things we wish we could do.

Every one of these influences plays a part in filling our void, and every one of them has an effect on the choices we make. This is how we become susceptible to brainwashing. Our parents may feed us well and make sure we go to bed at a sensible hour, but they also teach us that candy and late nights are special treats.

So we go through life valuing the benefits of sleep but valuing late nights even more; valuing a good diet but finding sugary and carb-laden foods hard to resist.

There's an old saying: everything is OK in moderation. But would you say that about heroin? We have to question these beliefs. Moderation implies a controlled amount that is not enough to do you any harm. But as I will explain, the way sugar, alcohol, nicotine, and stimulants work on the brain is to make you always want more. You don't really control these things at all—they control you.

Whichever way we are influenced by our role models, their influence overrides our natural instincts. In other words, we tend to do what we are told rather than what we feel. It is the clash between instinct and intellect. We will look at why this is in the coming chapters.

You might think that calling these influences "brainwashing" is a little extreme. After all, parents, teachers, friends, and other role models usually have our best interests at heart. They don't want to harm us or trick us into harming ourselves. But remember that all these role models have been brainwashed themselves, so while they pass on false information without realizing it, they pass it on nonetheless, and the brainwashing is all the more effective because it comes from a source we trust.

There is another influence we haven't mentioned—one that does attempt to trick us: the world of commerce. Commerce relies on people buying things they don't need, and businesses work very hard at persuading us that we do. Next time you watch TV, pay close attention to the ads. Can you honestly say you <u>need</u> any of the goods being pushed on you?

Sure, you might <u>want</u> that car, that perfume or that fast food, but the job of the advertiser is to make you think you <u>need</u> it, and they use highly persuasive means. You could call them illusions: the Illusion of Pleasure.

This, along with all the other influences in our lives, is what creates the Big Monster. So when it comes to making our own choices in life, the brainwashing, rather than natural instinct, takes over.

It is important to understand that these influences all have a negative impact on sleep because of the way they condition you to think. By trusting what we are told rather than our own natural instincts, we allow ourselves to be brainwashed into making bad lifestyle choices while convincing ourselves that we are choosing pleasure.

THE ILLUSION OF PLEASURE

When he was drafting the Declaration of Independence, Thomas Jefferson stated that among people's "unalienable rights" were "life, liberty and the pursuit of happiness." Which raises the question: What is happiness?

Pleasure certainly plays a part in the pursuit of happiness, but so do contentment, satisfaction, fulfillment, peace, and health. The pursuit of pleasure alone leads us into the trap. Smokers seek pleasure in cigarettes, but they never get satisfaction, never feel fulfilled. They become increasingly discontented, their minds are never at peace and their health suffers greatly. Any "pleasure" they think they get from the cigarette is illusory.

Human beings have become experts at creating the Illusion of Pleasure. It's how advertising works, along with all the other negative influences we are subjected to throughout our lives.

The human brain is easily tricked into detecting pleasure in things that are not only not pleasurable, but also harmful. Alcohol, nicotine, and other drugs, as well as fast food and other stimulants, contain chemicals that confuse, confound, and corrupt the brain's pleasure receptors. At the same time, we are told by role models and ads that these things are a source of pleasure—we are primed to expect genuine pleasure, so even though we feel an unease that follows the sense of pleasure created by a heady cocktail of that expectation, peer approval, sense of being rebellious, mature or part of a scene, the illusion becomes fixed and we start to crave that perceived "pleasure" again. Incidentally, the unease I mention is caused by withdrawal from the drug.

It is the Illusion of Pleasure that makes us pursue the bad lifestyle choices that have a harmful effect on sleep. That even includes choices like working extra hours and late nights. At the root of all these choices is the Illusion of Pleasure—the belief that our chosen action gives us some kind of benefit.

In the case of working late, the Illusion of Pleasure may be harder to identify but it is there. Perhaps it's the promise of making more money, or earning a promotion, or winning a contract, or just getting the boss off your back and buying some time further down the line. You might work late because you feel under pressure to do so, but retrace your steps—how did you come under such pressure? At the root of all these situations you will find a lifestyle choice.

It is the Illusion of Pleasure that makes us try to ease the effects of sleep loss by continuing to do the very things that cause it. We think we are in control of the choices we make, but we are not—the Big Monster is in control.

The Big Monster plays an ingenious trick. It convinces you, through the Illusion of Pleasure, that the only thing that can relieve your craving is the thing that caused it in the first place. Thus it guarantees that you remain trapped in a vicious circle—or a series of vicious circles—from which there is no escape as long as the Big Monster remains alive.

NO NEED TO MOPE

The process we are describing here is addiction. You might not like to think of yourself as an addict, and that's OK. The terms we use are not important—what matters is that you understand the process behind them. We will explain the cycle of addiction in the next chapter, and you can decide whether it applies to you—but in the meantime don't get bogged down with the word. The cause of your suffering is a subtle combination of brainwashing and misinformation creating addictive relationships with certain foods, drinks, and legal and / or illicit drugs, all leading to you making poor lifestyle choices based on phony, flawed information and triggers.

The word "addict" still tends to be associated with junkies, even though we know now that so many things in life are addictive—not just drugs, including nicotine and alcohol, but food additives like refined sugar, processed/starchy carbs, and even behaviors like gambling, shopping, and work. You might consider yourself to be slightly addicted or severely addicted— it's all the same trap. And if circumstances change, your addiction can go from slight to severe very quickly.

If that sounds like an attempt to frighten you out of your lifestyle choices and behaviors, that is not the intention at all. If it were that simple, those warnings on packs of cigarettes would scare everyone away from smoking for good. But they don't. The only place you see those warnings is in the hands of a cigarette smoker, and all they care about is the contents of the pack.

There is nothing to be afraid of because the solution is simple. You just need to kill the Big Monster. You do that by reversing all the brainwashing and seeing things as they really are—with your own senses.

The good news is that the brainwashing that has led to your behavior is reversible, and you don't have to go through any painful ordeal to achieve it. You just need to follow the instructions, step by step, and soon you will find your mindset beginning to change.

This is great news. There is no need to feel despondent any more. You have found a solution to your sleep problem, and there is nothing stopping you from achieving it. It is important that you take this on board and begin to look forward to a life free of insomnia.

Imagine how that will feel: looking forward to going to bed, knowing that you're going to get a good night's sleep, knowing that you'll wake up refreshed, restored, and re-energized. Now hold on to that thought.

The fourth instruction is:

Begin your journey, not with a feeling of doom and gloom, but with a feeling of elation. I have nothing but good news for you.

Chapter 5

ADDICTION

THE PITCHER PLANT

No one likes to be told they are not in control and that they have been fooled. Worse still, we don't like to feel we have lost control. Addicts will go into deep denial to kid themselves that they are in control of their drug. Any non-addict can clearly see that this is never the case.

Are we all addicts? That depends on your definition of addict. If the question is, "Are we all susceptible to the trap?" then the answer is yes.

Have you ever seen a pitcher plant—one of those carnivorous plants shaped like a tall jug, with digestive juices in the bottom? The pitcher plant feeds on flies, luring them in with the sweet smell of nectar and enticing them down beyond the point of no return.

When the fly first lands on the pitcher plant, it appears to be in control. It consumes the sweet nectar and moves around freely. But the fly always goes too far, wandering deeper into the trap until it loses its grip and falls into the belly of the plant.

There is a point at which the fly senses danger, as its feet lose their grip and it finds itself sliding down. But by this point it's too late. The fly is powerless to escape.

There are obvious comparisons between the pitcher plant and the addiction trap: the lure of perceived pleasure, the illusion of control, the feeling of helplessness when you realize you're in a trap, the continuous decline. This diagram illustrates it another way.

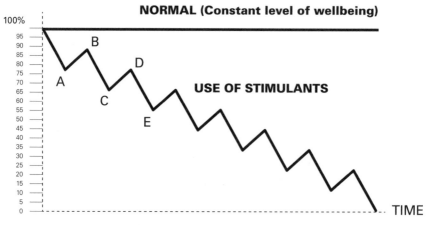

A CONTINUOUS DECLINE

With addiction, whether chemical or behavioral, the things you turn to for comfort take you further down while giving you the impression that they pick you up.

The pursuit of pleasure tempts us into behaviors that go against Mother Nature's guide. With regards to fatigue, we assume that our first use of a stimulant such as caffeine provides us with a genuine boost. The fact is, before we've even considered taking a sip of coffee, we've already fallen below the normal line—the line along which we are perfectly equipped to work, play, and rest. By ignoring Mother Nature's warning signs of fatigue, we end up moving downwards to the first point A. We are in an unnatural state of tiredness, we drink a shot of coffee, and experience that immediate boost upwards... not back to normal, just below (point B)—after all, we've now let a chemical stimulant into our body, but we feel better than we did a moment before. But all we're experiencing is the feeling of normality that we would have felt if we'd rested when prompted to by our body and brain. Gradually the caffeine withdraws from our body, and the feeling of fatigue returns and accompanies the mild, empty, insecure feeling caused by caffeine withdrawal, and we crash downwards to point C. We reach for something else that we believe will give us a boost—a sugary snack—and again we receive an immediate boost. We do feel better than we did a moment before—but the boost only takes us back to point D on the diagram... still not back to normal. Nonetheless, we are fooled into believing we've received a genuine boost before falling down again to point E... and so on. And so on. The more we experience this phony boost, the more we crave it when we're tired and run down. That craving is created by the manipulation of our blood-sugar levels, the impact of caffeine on our body and brain and the slight physical withdrawal (the Little Monster) combined with the ever-growing belief that the behavior or consumption does make us feel better—rather than realizing that each incident of use drags us deeper and deeper down into the pit of despair.

Artificial stimulants—caffeine, sugar etc—bombard your brain and body, akin to the high doses of fight-or-flight chemicals released when you sense danger. The brain is not designed to handle such high doses repeated over a sustained period, and in order to protect itself it builds a tolerance, just as rats build a tolerance to rat poison. As this occurs, we need more of the so-called stimulants to have an equal effect, which is why we consume more and more, but while doing so never getting back to normal—always experiencing what feels like a boost followed by a crash.

As you fall deeper into the trap, the highs become weaker and the lows become deeper. And so you go on, falling by ever-increasing amounts. You accelerate downwards. While each little boost continues to mislead you into believing that your stimulants are giving you some sort of pleasure or crutch, the reality is that you're becoming increasingly miserable and feeling dependent.

You can't deny it any more. You can see the effect that it is having on you and you feel confused and helpless at your inability to control it. We begin to accept this horrible existence as normal life. We never realize we should be cruising along feeling great; we spend all of our life in this downward spiral, with our sleep issue kicking in and turning a bad situation into a disaster zone.

We might attempt to fix our sleep issues from time to time with new pills, an early bedtime, homeopathic remedies, hypnotherapy, sleep apps, meditation and mindfulness. But while we continue to live our lives in this downward spiral behavior, our endeavors to change run out of steam and fall by the wayside. We accept this condition as being as good as life gets. No wonder you feel lousy!

REGAINING CONTROL

Most of us think we have no addictions. Or if we do, they are usually things we joke about: chocoholic, shopaholic, workaholic. We might call our lifestyle choices "vices," but we think we are in control of them, unlike those "poor junkies," we pity and regard as the real addicts.

It's only when you try to change that you realize you are not in control. Like the fly in the pitcher plant, it's the moment when you sense danger. It could be a health scare, a financial shock, the tired, prematurely old-looking face staring back at you from the mirror, or any other indicator that all is not well. Suddenly, you have a very good reason to change, but something keeps pulling you back in. That something is addiction—in the case of sleep issues, addiction to the foods, drinks, stimulants and behaviors that you think are the solution to your sleep problem when, in fact, they are either the cause or the exacerbators of the problem. You think you're in control of the problem—the fact is that it's the illusion of control.

The illusion of control is part of the ingenuity of the trap. The fly thinks it's in control as it gorges on nectar, but since it always turns out the same way, you have to ask whether the fly is ever really in control. If so, at what point does it lose control? When it loses its grip? Before that, perhaps, when it starts wandering in from the rim of the plant? In fact, the fly loses control the moment it lands on the plant. It has already fallen for the trap.

We may feel in control when we first start smoking or drinking or gambling, or any of the other sleep-disruptive lifestyle choices that we perceive as pleasure, but the diagram shows that this is not the case. We hand over control to the drug the first time we take it, and we lose control the further into the trap we fall. At any point below normality in your descent, you are relinquishing control to the Big Monster.

The fight against sleep encompasses many such traps. Despite the many obvious comparisons with the pitcher plant, however, there is one essential difference. Unlike the fly, you can escape any time you want. The fly never understands the nature of the trap it's in, but you can. To do so, it's important that you first recognize the traps you're in and acknowledge that you are not completely in control. If you could talk to the fly, you would tell it to stop feeding while it is still in a position to escape. You are in a position to escape any time you want—and that is what you're ready to do by the time you finish this book.

Understanding the steps you have to take in order to break free from the issues that interfere with your sleep is actually quite liberating. And that, in turn, will help you regain control.

Being controlled is like being in the middle of a tug-of-war. Pulling you one way is the knowledge that your way of life is not helping you solve your sleep problem; pulling the opposite way is the fear that changing your way of life will involve sacrifices that you don't want to make. As you begin to regain control, you will start to see that these are not sacrifices but positive choices that bring only benefits. So, remembering the fourth instruction—to begin your journey with a feeling of elation—let's start addressing those lifestyle choices that are disrupting your sleep.

It's time to take those first steps to freedom.

Chapter 6

FIRST STEPS TO FREEDOM

•REMOVE THE ILLUSIONS •THE REAL REASON YOU CAN'T SLEEP •IDENTIFY YOUR ADDICTIONS •RETHINK YOUR LIFESTYLE CHOICES

REMOVE THE ILLUSIONS

The Illusion of Pleasure lies behind most, if not all, of the bad choices we make in life. These choices are influenced by role models and advertising. Today, the widespread addiction to social media makes it even easier for advertisers to brainwash us into behaviors that are not good for us.

The first step to freedom is to recognize this state of affairs.

In order to cure your insomnia, you first need to change your mindset—both toward sleep and toward the multitude of lifestyle factors that affect it. That change of mindset begins by recognizing and acknowledging that many of the "pleasures" you seek day-to-day are actually illusions, which have been peddled to you by people with a vested interested in keeping you hooked.

If you think that sounds ridiculously simple, that's because it is. The truth is, we go through life absorbing influences from all directions and rarely, if ever, question them. Have you ever questioned whether chocolate really tastes good? Have you ever challenged the belief that drinking alcohol helps you relax and have fun?

Smokers believe all kinds of myths about nicotine and cigarettes.

They help you relax.

They help you concentrate.

They give you confidence.

They calm you down.

Etc

Many of these myths even contradict each other, but smokers go through their smoking lives believing all of them and, worse, believing life will be a miserable mess without all these things if they quit.

They somehow overlook the fact that their lives are a miserable mess because they smoke.

We don't question these myths, because we are never told to.

So here's the fifth instruction:

Question everything you think you know about sleep, addiction, and behavior.

I also want you to scrutinize everything you read here, too, because only then can you truly determine what is true and what is false. You will find, upon examination, that everything you read in this book makes complete sense.

DON'T PANIC!

In order to solve your problem with sleep you're not going to be asked to stop drinking alcohol, stop using your smartphone, stop drinking coffee or stop eating refined sugar or processed/starchy carbs. The fact is, when you turn your mind to it, you should be able to adapt your lifestyle and your food and drink consumption with ease, in spite of any sense of reliance you have on those foods, drinks, and activities. For those who feel they want to go further and eliminate them, or somehow struggle to do so, Easyway provides a specific program for all of those issues, and others.

When you stop and question the myths that keep you in the trap, it's like a light switching on in your mind. You immediately start seeing things differently. Here's an exercise that highlights the point.

MINDFUL EATING

What's your favorite treat? Cake? Cookies? Candy bars? Whenever you give yourself this treat, your brain anticipates the pleasure in advance. In other words, you're convinced that it's going to be delicious before you put it anywhere near your mouth.

Now let's challenge that. Use your senses to get the full effect of your favorite treat.

Now look at that treat closely. Whatever it is—cake, cookies, ice cream, chocolate—does it look delicious?

Examine the color and texture slowly. Now hold it to your nose. How does it smell? Does it smell like anything? Does it have an appealing aroma? Does it smell a little synthetic, or does it smell natural?

Take a bite, but don't just chew it up and swallow it. Hold it in your mouth. Be aware of how it feels. Is it chewy or crunchy? Does it turn to mush in your mouth? And how does it taste? How would you describe the flavor?

When you finish, how satisfied do you feel? Has it left you feeling energized and healthy? Has the craving gone, or are you craving more? Does a part of you wish you hadn't eaten it?

Eating in this mindful way can completely change your perception of certain foods. The reason is that we don't usually pay attention to these sensory aspects of the foods that we regard as our favorites. Their appeal lies almost entirely in our minds. We anticipate the pleasure, and when we eat the food we temporarily satisfy that anticipation.

But it doesn't last. That's how you can tell the difference between genuine and illusory satisfaction. The latter quickly passes and is followed by a craving.

When you do pay attention to how foods look, smell, feel and taste, you get a better perception of the foods that are good to eat and the foods that aren't.

A blueberry, a raspberry, a strawberry, or an apple, for example, all have a wonderful aroma, a beautiful color and texture, they feel fresh or crisp in the mouth, and they taste naturally sweet and delicious.

How far we've strayed from that sense of natural eating. We even have to be wary of some fruit, as these days some—normally marked "extra sweet"—have been genetically or synthetically modified to enhance their level of sweetness. This is done because so little attention has been paid to growing the fruit correctly, in accordance with the seasons and with care. A lot of modern farming has focused on getting the produce all the same shape, the same color, the same size, the same flavor regardless of ripeness, and delivered with the maximum shelf life.

Challenging everything you have believed to be true up to this point in your life is the only way to unravel the illusions that keep you trapped in cycles of behavior that are disastrous for sleep.

Overleaf is another exercise to illustrate how your mindset changes in an instant when you look more carefully.

Take a look at the different-sized coffee cups in the picture over the page.

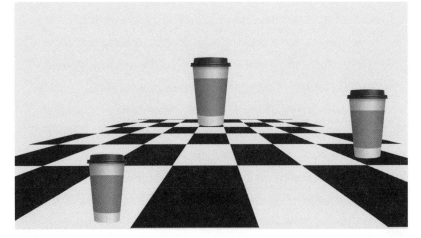

If someone told you they're all the same size, you would question their judgment, wouldn't you? You've already accepted that they're different sizes because that's what I told you and that's what you see.

Nevertheless, the fact is, they're all exactly the same size. Look again. Still skeptical? Take a ruler and measure them. Surprising, isn't it?

This illustrates how easy it is to change your mindset when presented with the full set of facts. So let's apply this to some of the causes of insomnia.

THE REAL REASON YOU CAN'T SLEEP

For the chronic insomniac, the trap can feel like a prison from which you can never escape. This can bring about a feeling of resignation. You blame yourself and feel doomed to a life of sleepless misery. There hardly seems to be any point in trying any more.

But when you understand the nature of the trap you're in and how it twists your perception of reality, you begin to see that there is a way out. The reason you can't sleep is not because of the way you are made or because of the life fate has handed you; it's because you have been brainwashed into making certain lifestyle choices that are not conducive to sleep, and maintained them in spite of your better judgment. The motivation for the latter is based on false evidence, that you'll enjoy life less if you're forced to make a change. No one is going to force you to do anything. There's a big difference between feeling shoehorned into doing something and happily deciding to change certain behaviors to achieve a huge bonus.

The next step is to identify these choices and behaviors and change them.

Recognizing that you have been brainwashed changes your whole way of looking at the problem. For the first time, you can see that it's not a weakness in you that makes you suffer from insomnia, and the feeling of powerlessness and resignation goes. You realize that escape is within reach. All you have to do is make different choices.

Say that to a smoker and they will snigger with disdain. "Sure, I'll just choose to stop smoking. Easy."

This response reveals two important points: 1, that all smokers wish they could stop; 2, that making different choices is not easy when you have the Big Monster in your brain.

Smokers constantly try to quit but keep getting dragged back into the trap. Why? Because they can't shake the belief that smoking gives them some sort of pleasure or crutch. In other words, they fear that they won't be able to cope without their drug.

The same belief applies to all addicts—and addiction goes far beyond the acknowledged drugs, like nicotine, alcohol, heroin and cocaine. We can get addicted to other substances, like sugar and caffeine, and to activities like gambling, social media and even shopping.

How many of these substances and behaviors play a part in your lifestyle? The real reason you can't sleep is because you are not allowing yourself to, due to lifestyle choices that might have developed into early-stage addictions.

IDENTIFY YOUR ADDICTIONS

Every type of addiction works in the same way. The drug or activity disrupts the brain's normal functions, causing the victim to lose sight of genuine pleasures in favor of phony ones. Gambling is a good example that doesn't involve taking a drug. As children, we expend huge amounts of energy over long periods of time. Put a bunch of kids in a playground with a ball, anywhere in the world, and they'll start throwing it or kicking it around. Left to their own devices, kids will play soccer for hours on end, just for the sheer fun of it—win or lose. Having said that, make no mistake, these games are highly competitive.

It's in our nature. Young kids will race each other to the nearest gate, lamppost, or fence. They revel in it. Can you see how that sense of fun becomes grotesquely distorted the first time one of the kids suggests a bet? "$1 in! First one to the reach the fence wins!" Something that was pure, genuine, fun—win or lose—suddenly becomes serious. This immediately begins to interfere with the way the kids' brains perceive not only victory and defeat, but simply taking part. The high of winning is no different—it's the sense of foreboding, risk, and jeopardy in the buildup that is amplified—as are the pain and misery of defeat. These are new levels of adrenaline highs and lows, and unlike the caveman who only experienced those levels of intense jeopardy in the avoidance of saber-toothed tigers, the child begins to live with it as normal background "noise."

Something that was normal, healthy and fun—win, lose, or draw—has suddenly become a source of angst and gloom. Can you see how, having tasted bitter defeat in the "$ race," a child's sense of victory would appear that much greater than a victory before its invention, simply because the joy of taking part has become diminished and corrupted? The feeling of victory isn't greater—but we buy into the illusion.

All addictive drugs behave in a similar way to disrupt our ability to identify genuine pleasure versus illusory pleasure.

We're brainwashed by fiction, Hollywood, and rock stars to believe that illicit and legal drugs provide us with a genuine high—so we're already predisposed to that idea. But if a child with no knowledge whatsoever of, for example, cocaine, were to be given the drug without their knowledge, they would report feeling unwell and would need to be cared for until they felt better.

Of course, the first shot of the drug is also tied up in the emotion of the moment, the peer approval, the rebelliousness, the sheer sense of glamour or of forbidden fruit, and it's easy to mistake that, combined with the physical and mental effects of the drug, for a genuine high.

As the drug wears off, it withdraws from the body, and for the first time the person experiences a low—like a void. It wasn't there before the first shot of the drug—it didn't exist—but it's there now. When the drug is reintroduced to the body, that void, that low, is replaced and the addict feels better than they did a moment before—they are fooled into thinking that the drug has provided relief when, in fact, it has merely temporarily relieved the void, the low, that it created.

Whether you're a drug user or not, a gambler or not, I don't expect the "$ game" anecdote or the above paragraphs to convince you that you get no genuine pleasure from it; it would take a few more hours of specialized Easyway attention to achieve that. But hopefully you can understand in principle how drug addicts, or those suffering from behavioral issues, are fooled into thinking they get a high from their drug or behavior when in fact they do not.

There is a lot of concern about kids and their addiction to their phones. Try taking their phone away and see how they respond. It's like taking away a junkie's stash.

You might think this is going too far. You're not a junkie. You don't think you're addicted to anything, even mildly. OK, so how would you feel if someone took away your phone, or a piece of cake you've just cut, or a cookie you'd saved for later, or your first alcoholic drink of the evening, or your pack of cigarettes, or whatever your personal "treat" may be?

If you're honest with yourself, you'd no doubt expect to be extremely unhappy. Can you imagine feeling the same if someone beat you to the last few Brussels sprouts at the dinner table? Probably not. It's the behavior, food, drinks, and drugs that create a dramatic swing in mood when we are not allowed them that are prone to inspire addiction and addictive behavior.

You're going to break free from your sleep issue. All you need to do is make a few simple changes in your life, follow the instructions in this book and look forward to freedom rather than anticipate problems.

Addiction is rife, although it affects different people to different degrees. That is not because of the way different people are made; it's because the influences we are exposed to are all different and come at different times and in different circumstances.

Most of us manage our addictions quite comfortably… until we have to go without them or we suffer from some associated health problem. Think about diets. Most diets require you to go without the foods you hold dear. They involve sacrifice, willpower, and a lot of misery. Nobody finds it easy. As soon as you hit your target weight, do you continue with the diet? No, you go right back to the junk food and your weight springs back up, usually higher than when you started.

Your mindset regarding those foods has not changed. In fact, if anything, you become more addicted because the dieting process reinforces the belief that you can't enjoy life without them.

In order to empower yourself to make different lifestyle choices, you have to change your mindset. You have to unravel the brainwashing that creates the desire for these things and see the true picture—that these things do nothing for you whatsoever.

If you need more help in overcoming any specific addiction, you will find that the range of Allen Carr Easyway books covers most of them and will take you through the method in detail for that addiction. Insomnia is not itself an addiction, but it can be caused by any or all of the common addictions, from smoking to gambling to overeating to digital devices.

As long as you continue to make what you believe to be lifestyle choices and they continue to control you, you will not be helping your chances of getting a good night's sleep. The aim is to put your mind and body in the state intended by Mother Nature's guide, so sleep comes naturally and brings you all the necessary benefits.

That doesn't mean you have to live in a cave with no electronic devices and eat berries for the rest of your life (although you would probably sleep very well if you did); you just need to develop an awareness of these choices and how they control you, and reverse the brainwashing so you control them.

As we mentioned at the beginning, tech devices are fantastic tools that can make life a whole lot easier and more fun—but scrolling frenetically for fear of missing out just before you go to bed is not a sign of being in control!

RETHINK YOUR LIFESTYLE CHOICES

The biggest thing that makes anyone rethink their lifestyle choices is a health scare. A heart attack, a stroke, the onset of type 2 diabetes, hypertension, cancer… These are frightening words that can jolt us into a change of mindset. It's time to add insomnia to that list.

Losing sleep is not just a threat to your health and wellbeing for the next day or the day after, it is proven to be a forewarning of serious health conditions like Parkinson's disease and Alzheimer's many years later.

Aren't we lucky? Mother Nature gives us this warning sign. Wouldn't it be crazy to ignore it?!

So take some time to examine the aspects of your lifestyle that might be sabotaging your sleep. Re-read Chapter 3 if you need prompting as to what some of these aspects may be. When you start to really scrutinize your choices, as in the mindful eating exercise, you get a strong sense of what is good for you and what isn't, what you have control over and what you don't.

Once you have identified the behaviors that could be controlling you and disrupting your sleep, make a plan to change them. Read the relevant Allen Carr Easyway book if it's an addiction you need help in quitting.

The aim is to examine what you currently believe to be true and question it in every detail. For example, say you drink alcohol frequently because you believe it helps you relax, makes you more lively company and generally leads to you having a good time. Ask yourself,

"Does it really help me relax, or does it make me feel a little uptight and irritable, especially the next day?"

"Does it really make me more lively company, or does it blind me to my real behavior, which can be kind of embarrassing?"

"Does it really help me to have a good time, or is that all about the occasion and the company?"

Question everything, challenge all your beliefs, and notice how your mindset starts to change. This is the process of killing the Big Monster. Once the Big Monster is dead, it becomes easy to change your lifestyle choices because there is no desire to fight. You don't need willpower. There is no feeling of deprivation, no discomfort or misery, only the elation of knowing you are restoring yourself to the wonderful condition that Mother Nature intended.

Chapter 7

THE INCREDIBLE MACHINE

Let's recap what we have established so far. Sleep is a vital process during which mind and body are cleansed of toxins, cells are restored and new growth occurs, and sensory experiences are saved, processed, and analyzed.

Insufficient sleep has an immediate effect on performance, judgment, and mood and is a warning sign of critical health issues to come many years down the line.

We are not programmed to suffer from insomnia. It occurs as a consequence of certain lifestyle choices, which flood the mind with natural or unnatural chemicals that counteract our natural sleep processes.

These are choices we make as individuals, but we do not make them freely. They are influenced by role models, advertising, and addictions, so we regard them as normal, natural choices. But when you stop and question the brainwashing, you begin to see that these choices are far from natural.

It's at this point in the method that doubts can start to creep in.

"Are you saying I have to give up all my pleasures in life?"
"I don't want to change my whole lifestyle! I just need some sleep!"

Rest assured, you are not expected to "give up" anything, nor to sacrifice any pleasures. On the contrary, the purpose of Easyway is to help people live a happier, healthier life, not make them suffer.

But ask yourself this: would you respond like that if a doctor told you that you had a serious heart condition? OK, some people do. They keep drinking and smoking and eating junk because they say they would rather live a "full life" than live forever depriving themselves.

When the heart attack comes, they wish they could turn back time. But they have missed the point. Living with a serious health problem is not living a full life. And, as we have established, insomnia is a serious health problem. If you have any doubts about this, go back and re-read Chapter 2.

The more sensible heart patients listen to their doctor's advice and change their lifestyle. What they discover is not a life of deprivation and misery but a newfound vigor, clear-headedness and a more positive outlook—especially if they use Easyway to achieve it. It's exactly what nature intended.

Because of the brainwashing, we dismiss the lifestyle choices that nature has designed for us. Instead, we embrace self-destructive behaviors and convince ourselves that they give us pleasure, even when we know deep down that they do the complete opposite.

USER'S MANUAL—WARNING SIGNS

The car is a very sophisticated piece of machinery with lots of moving parts and electrical circuits, all of which need attention from time to time. So car manufacturers equip their products with a warning system. If your oil is low, a light comes on. If there is not enough air in your tires, a different light comes on. If the engine is overheating, another light comes on. Etc etc.

If you're not sure what the light means, you have the User's Manual to tell you. You look it up, find out what the fault is, and do something to fix it.

The human body is an even more sophisticated machine than the car and it, too, has a warning system that sends you a clear signal when something is wrong. It's called pain, and there is no need for a User's Manual—pain tells us exactly where the problem is, and how severe.

There are many levels of pain, from the mild discomfort you feel after a bad night's sleep to excruciating agony. To avoid the former developing into the latter, it's advisable to take action promptly.

But instead of regarding pain as a valuable survival function, we treat it as an unnecessary evil and take drugs to numb it. Imagine if the oil warning light came on in your car and instead of adding oil you applied a piece of tape so you could no longer see the light. Sure, you'd get rid of the warning light, but you would soon say goodbye to your car, too. Yet that's exactly what we do when we take painkillers. Rather than addressing the source of the problem, we knock out the warning light.

Your senses are also part of that early warning system. Sight, smell, touch, and taste all play a part in detecting poison. Watch a cat approach food. First, they will look at it from a safe distance, then they will go up and sniff it. They might prod it with a paw and then, if all these senses are satisfied, they will taste it, tentatively at first.

Your senses do the same for you. You can tell when an apple is rotten by looking at it. If it's going bad, it might look edible but it will smell funny and will be soft to the touch. If you took a bite, the taste would be putrid and you would spit it out. An experience like that might keep you away from apples for a while. There is no one pressurizing you to persevere.

Your senses try to protect you when you first drink alcohol or smoke a cigarette. No one likes the smell or taste at first. Often it makes them sick. This is the body's protection system first trying to prevent the taking of poison and then trying to expel it. It's ingenious. Yet we think we know better, and we try the poison again and again, until we build up a tolerance to it.

We call this "acquiring the taste." We are actually acquiring a loss of taste.

THE FLAW IN THE INCREDIBLE MACHINE

Human beings inflict suffering on themselves in ways that the rest of the animal kingdom does not. You don't see wild animals with drug addictions, suffering from obesity or insomnia, so how come humans, the most intelligent species on the planet, fall victim to so many self-inflicted ailments?

The clue lies in the word "intelligent." The key difference between human beings and wild animals is that animals survive solely by instinct. The only ones who do not are those whose diets are controlled by humans (pets), and those whose instincts become corrupted by feeding on our (largely) addictive food waste (pests). Humans also use instinct to survive, but the tool that has enabled us to rule over the animal kingdom is intellect.

Our intellect has given us the capacity to learn and pass on our learning; the result is that we have developed into a highly sophisticated species that is not only capable of building fantastic structures and machines, but also has an appreciation of art, music, romance, spirituality, and so on. Intellect is a wonderful thing, but it can go to your head; for it is our intellect that has also led us astray.

Rather than building on the advantage that Mother Nature has given us, to live peaceful, healthy, happy lives, we have devoted a remarkable amount of time to self-destruction—not just in the ever more sophisticated ways of killing each other, but in the way we abuse our bodies and minds.

By allowing our intellect to override our instincts, we have become a species of anxious, stressed-out, tired, junk-food consumers and drug addicts. Instinct is Mother Nature's survival kit. It tells us when and what to eat, it alerts us to danger, it even helps us find a suitable mate. But there are times when it conflicts with our intellect, and then we tend to trust the lessons we've been told over our instincts. Why? Because instinct often gives us the answer we don't want to hear.

It's precisely this conflict that raises doubts in the method. The thought that you might need to change aspects of your lifestyle clashes with your intellectual belief that these are all things that make you happy.

Our tendency to trust intellectual opinion over and above our own instincts is the flaw in the human machine. When we make intellectual choices based on misinformation—like drinking alcohol to help us cope with stress—our wellbeing suffers.

Intellect can cause great happiness and it can cause extreme misery. The choice is ours. So why do we so often take the self-destructive option? Quite simply,

WE DON'T ALWAYS REALIZE WE HAVE AN OPTION.

HOW WE ARE BRAINWASHED

Brainwashing might strike you as an excessively strong word. It smacks of spy novels, evil regimes, and *Nineteen Eighty-Four*'s Big Brother. No one likes the thought that they are being brainwashed, and we find it hard to accept. But thanks to recent exposés of the tactics used by social media platforms, we are now more aware than ever that we are very susceptible to being manipulated and controlled by other humans without even realizing it.

This isn't some wacky conspiracy theory. These are the everyday forces of commerce and power at work. The power of persuasion. Advertisers have done it for decades, and they're not the only ones. We do it to one another.

The reason human beings suffer so many self-inflicted ailments is because there are always other human beings who stand to gain as a result of those destructive behaviors. We all revile the drug dealer who gives children free drugs in the playground to get them hooked into buying more later, but it's the same business model that earns billions for many so-called "respectable" companies. Freebies up front, premium prices later, when we're hooked.

We walk blindly into the trap because we think we love those freebies. We believe they are going to make us happier.

Nobody chooses to become an addict for the rest of their life. No one has that first drink thinking, "Great! I'm on my way to becoming an alcoholic." We have it because we think it is the thing to do. The manufacturers don't even have to persuade us; we persuade each other.

We are pressured into these self-destructive behaviors by society, by our peers, by our role models, and by our own beliefs, formed by years of brainwashing. In the face of such pressure, is it any surprise that so many of us find ourselves in a trap?

UNRAVELING THE ILLUSIONS

There are essentially two myths that lead us into the trap and keep us there:

1. The myth that drinking, smoking, eating junk food, gambling, and burning the candle at both ends gives you pleasure or a crutch.

2. The myth that stopping or changing our behavior will be hard and leave us feeling miserable.

Now, with all this talk of brainwashing, you might be thinking, How do I know that Easyway isn't just trying to brainwash me, too? By all means ask that question—and keep asking it. The more you question, the more clearly you will see the truth.

The brainwashing we're exposed to from birth, by loved ones, society in general, TV, movies, the food and drink industry, and our brains being fooled into valuing illusory pleasures by our descent into a variety of addictions or addictive behaviors is like the gradual tightening of a spring. It gets tighter and tighter and tighter and approaches the "breaking point." What Easyway does is effectively, gently, gradually, and sensitively loosen that coiled spring, little by little, until eventually it returns to its original form. Easyway is counter-brainwashing—never forget that.

There is one surefire way to get to the truth. Use your senses and instincts and follow the third instruction: Reject anything that goes against Mother Nature's guide.

If you practiced the mindful eating exercise in the last chapter, you had a taste (literally) of the power of your senses and instincts to override the brainwashing when you take the trouble to connect with them. By applying this method to all the so-called pleasures that impact negatively on sleep, you will start to unravel the first myth.

Challenge your "pleasures" with the following questions:

Does it really taste great?

Do I really like the smell?

Does it really feel good?

Does it really give me confidence?

Do I really feel more relaxed?

Is it really helping me concentrate?

Is it really making me more entertaining/interesting?

Am I really enjoying this?

Or…

Am I confusing the belief that it feels/tastes/smells great with the temporary boost of getting my fix?

Am I confusing a sense of relaxation with the temporary relief of ending my craving?

Am I confusing heightened concentration with the removal of the distraction of withdrawal or craving?

Am I confusing self-confidence with a loss of self-awareness?

Remember, this is all aimed at helping you get the sleep you need. As you ask these questions, you will start to see through the illusions, and your attitude to making different lifestyle choices will change. You will no longer see it as a sacrifice.

The genius of the Incredible Machine is that it is designed to guide us toward genuine pleasures. Real happiness is being in tune with your instincts. When you ask the questions, when you pay close attention to your sensory responses, you quickly see and feel that this is true.

It sounds ridiculously simple—and it is. What is more ridiculous is that other methods complicate it. We go through life without ever asking these questions. Why? Because no one tells us to. That is where Easyway is different. And it's why Easyway has been so successful at helping people overcome their self-destructive behaviors where other methods have repeatedly failed. So far, it's estimated to have helped more than 50 million people worldwide.

Chapter 8

ANXIETY

•WHY WE GET ANXIOUS •WHY OUR ANCESTORS WERE
ABLE TO SLEEP SOUNDLY •CAUSES OF CHRONIC ANXIETY
•CHOOSING CALM

So far, we have established that there are lifestyle choices we make that disrupt our sleep—and in order to get back to a regular, natural sleep pattern, you need to change some or all of those choices. But there is another factor that is also hugely disruptive to sleep, over which we seem to have no choice: anxiety.

Anxiety is a major barrier to sleep. And it is one of the most powerful of all the vicious circles.

As long as you feel anxious you will not be able to sleep, because the very purpose of anxiety is to keep you alert.

WHY WE GET ANXIOUS

Anxiety is nothing to be ashamed of. It is wired into our DNA for the very good reason that it is crucial to our survival. When faced with a threat, our muscles tense, our heart rate increases and our breathing becomes shorter and more intense. These physical responses are all designed to prepare us for fight or flight—to tackle our assailant or to run away.

We know these physical responses as fear. Anxiety is the part of the fear instinct that prepares us for potential threats.

In other words, the things we get anxious about are not immediate threats that we have to deal with there and then; they are imagined or potential threats. That is not to say the anxiety is unnecessary. If you're walking down a dark alley at night, the anxiety you feel is preparing you for the possibility of someone attacking you. There is no immediate threat. You're not being confronted by an assailant; you're responding to the possibility that it could happen. And even though you know it's a rare occurrence, it is still a possibility, and you need to be prepared.

The ability to foresee potential dangers is not an intellectual faculty. Wild animals have it too. If an antelope senses that a lion may be present, it stops grazing and tenses up, its eyes start scanning, its nose and ears twitch to pick up scents and sounds that might tell it where the lion is. It can't see the lion, it is not under immediate attack, but it can sense that an attack might be coming and it prepares. When the lion breaks cover, the antelope is ready to spring away, like a sprinter in the "set" position on the blocks. In most cases, the antelope survives.

Anxiety is an essential survival instinct. Our hunter-gatherer ancestors relied on it every day, just as an antelope relies on it every day. But our ancestors didn't suffer from insomnia like we do. Why?

WHY OUR ANCESTORS WERE
ABLE TO SLEEP SOUNDLY

Our ability to imagine dangers is a natural instinct hard-wired into our DNA, but it has also become an intellectual faculty. We can create anxiety where there is no threat to our survival.

Sometimes we do this for entertainment. A fairground ride, a horror movie; we know how to create fear without real danger. Even though we know that there is no danger, the suggestion of danger is enough to trigger the instinct of fear.

Why do we choose to frighten ourselves? Because the natural reaction is exhilarating. We are put on high alert, we get an adrenaline rush, a thrill. But this rush is only designed to last long enough for us to run or fight. Overdo it and mind and body begin to suffer.

We are not designed to live with frequent bombardments of stimulation triggering prolonged adrenaline rushes. We can deal with a scary movie without too much trouble—but can you imagine the impact that the constant overstimulation of online gaming or social media has on our minds and bodies?

In 2022, one of the most emotionally hostile "places" on earth was the Twitter social media platform. Millions of people were getting angry with others whose opinions differed. More than that, the unbridled anger and aggression were unleashed digitally; constant disagreement, constant indiscriminate verbal attacks, vile behavior, with all involved drunk on a heady brew of pious self-righteousness, convinced that they were right and that they were fighting some kind of online battle between good and evil.

Nuance, politeness, restraint, and understanding that someone else may have an entirely different view from your own, yet perhaps you both could be right, all went by the wayside. A smartalecky, cutting reply, seemingly trumping any attempt at making a constructive, considered assessment of another's point of view.

This was where unrestricted, unbridled, constant over-stimulation took us.

Social media? More like antisocial media!

Twitter is just one example of modern life that promised so much, but became hamstrung through a large minority of its users riding a cheap-thrill, adrenaline-fueled descent into the utter chaos of "punch first, ask questions later" online aggression.

In fact, it's the distant, largely anonymous, protected online nature of the discourse that has turned it into such a toxic "battlefield." If these people behaved this way face to face, in accordance with even the most modern version of the laws of the jungle, they would very quickly come to great physical harm. To avoid that, instinctively sensing the potential danger through a level of genuine anxiety, they would use discretion, understanding, and open discussion to reach an agreement, or to simply agree to disagree.

In the "Twittersphere," it was the absence of genuine self-protecting anxiety, and the excess of adrenaline, that created such a horrible environment.

Ironically, the end result for those involved is fatigue, dissatisfaction, and stress leading to depression and anxiety, all combining to create the perfect conditions for a sleep problem.

In all but a few users, no minds have been changed and no positive or useful action achieved. All in return for the momentary "thrill" of a few "likes," retweets, and comments from people you've never met. Can you see how empty and shallow the so-called thrill I mention above truly is? It's like wearing shoes that are too tight just for the relief of taking them off. Pointless and painful.

Other anxieties brought on by intellectual reasoning also help us survive—or at least avoid threats—but these anxieties can set in long-term, and that's when they, too, can disrupt sleep.

The fears associated with losing your job, for example, are intellectual. You have learned about the possible consequences of finding yourself unemployed—e.g. having no money, being forced to sell your possessions, sacrificing the pleasures and comforts you enjoy, feeling worthless and unfulfilled—so you do everything you can to protect your job and make yourself indispensable, even when there is no threat of losing your job.

You can't dispute the reasoning behind wanting to keep your job, but if job security becomes a long-term source of anxiety, it will disrupt your sleep.

Chronic anxiety is symptomatic of the way we live today. We perceive threats in many different situations and we get stuck with them. Our ancestors did not suffer from such chronic anxieties, so they were able to sleep soundly at night, even though the threats to their survival were much more real and numerous than anything we encounter.

CAUSES OF CHRONIC ANXIETY

When we talk about chronic anxiety, we mean any anxiety that lasts longer than the short burst designed to prepare us for fight or flight. Anything that threatens us is a cause of anxiety. For our hunter-gatherer ancestors, those threats would be hunger, thirst, cold, illness, natural disaster, and physical attack. As social beings, they may have experienced some anxiety as to their place in the tribe or their mating instinct. But they would not have endured many of the chronic anxieties that plague us today.

Anxieties such as:

Money

Money is a man-made source of anxiety. Some of us desire it more than others, but whatever your attitude to money, it's virtually impossible to live in the so-called civilized world without it. If you want a home, heat, running water, electricity, or food, you need money. And these are just the basics.

As we acquire more money, we open up more choices, all of which require even more money: cars, restaurants, vacations, entertainment, hobbies, schools, clothes, phones, watches, TVs, jewelry, furniture...

To be clear, there is absolutely nothing wrong with spending money on things that give you pleasure or make life easier. It becomes a problem when you feel pressured into buying things, because when you start to feel that money is running out, or you don't have enough for the things you think you need, your imagination flies to the thought of not even being able to afford the basics and anxiety kicks in. You see homeless people, and you hear stories of how quickly people can lose everything, and the thought of that happening to you is frightening. So money anxiety is a sleep disruptor that affects most people at some time in their life.

Work

Because work is our main source of income, it is closely tied to money anxiety. The threat of losing your job means the threat of having no income. But there are other anxieties associated with work that can torment you in the middle of the night.

Impostor syndrome—the fear of being found to be lacking in the skills that people assume you have—is a common anxiety. "Will I meet the boss's expectations?" "Will I be shown up in front of my team?" "Are they planning to get rid of me?" It's not just the fear of losing your income—it's also the fear of embarrassment and the sense of shame.

Of course, there really isn't any shame or embarrassment in losing your job—everyone around you will feel nothing but goodwill and positive vibes for you—but our fear of it persists, driven mainly by the fear of our lives being turned upside down.

There might be absolutely no basis for these anxieties. You could be getting glowing reports from your superiors, but still imagine that there is some alternative story going on behind what you see with your own eyes.

Another major source of anxiety when it comes to work is time—or lack of it. "This is going to take two days, but the client wants it tomorrow." Like money, time is a man-made concept that always seems to be in short supply. Our early *Homo sapiens* ancestors didn't worry about being time-poor. They didn't have alarm clocks or watches or calendars or deadlines. They lived by the sun and adapted to the seasons—and they slept soundly at night.

Relationships

Our ancestors did have relationships, and they might have worried about their partner's feelings, but relationships these days are made more complicated by the weight of expectation.

TV, movies, and social media feed us images of what the perfect relationship should look like, and it's easy to feel we're failing somehow if our relationships do not replicate what we see on screen. Of course, what we see on screen is a fantasy, but that doesn't stop us from believing in it.

So we look for signs that our relationships match the fantasy, question our expectations, fret about things rather than enjoying the moment, perhaps feeling that we, our lives, our reality, are somehow inadequate.

Relationship anxiety goes beyond your relationship with your partner. You can have relationship problems with a family member or a friend, or even someone you don't really know. A small disagreement with a stranger in a store will cause anxiety, because there is the immediate threat of a confrontation and then there is the perceived threat of social disapproval. "Should I have said that?" "Did I embarrass myself?" "Should I have been more mature?" "Did I let them get the better of me?" Social anxiety begins in the schoolyard and continues through life. We want to be accepted. We want to belong. If we don't, it makes us feel vulnerable and that triggers the survival instinct.

Thanks to social media, social anxiety is more common than ever. We look to our devices for signs of approval. How many followers? How many likes? What did they mean by that comment? Social media has generated a new syndrome—fear of missing out (FOMO). Thanks to social media, it is very easy to be cruel, and it is equally easy to misread other people's meanings. We perceive social disapproval where it doesn't exist.

Social media has also put our relationships on the world stage, so a disagreement that might have resulted in a nasty comment in the playground can now blow up for thousands or—in the case of some celebrities—millions to see. The stakes are very high, and the price of getting it wrong can be terrifying.

Nerves

In our pursuit of fun, respect, or to make the world a better place, we put ourselves in situations that make us nervous. A big competition, a performance, a public-speaking engagement, a responsible position in a community club, a PTA role, a team sport... We don't have to do these things. They are not essential for our survival. But there is a lot to gain from doing them.

Nevertheless, the level of nerves is not always proportional to the prize. That's because our anxiety is not just about failing to win, or delivering success, or maintaining standards. It's about the social price of failure. "What will people say?" "How will they react?" And we start to doubt our own ability or even our right to be in that situation. It's these anxieties that lead the majority of people to avoid getting involved in such roles. The attitude is, "Why should I get involved? Somebody else can put their neck on the line."

Children

Our ancient ancestors would certainly have worried about their children from time to time. The nurturing instinct would have given them concern if their children became ill, were injured, or got cornered by a wild animal. But today parents have many more anxieties to keep them awake at night.

"Are they happy enough?" "Are they healthy enough?" "Are they popular enough?" "Are they being bullied?" "Are they bullying?" "Are they talented enough?" "Are they confident enough?" "Are they on track at school?" "Are they actually going to school?" "Will they make the team?" "How will I manage their disappointment if they don't?" "How long are they spending on that game?" "Is their girlfriend/boyfriend right for them?" "What time are they coming home?" "What if they're using drugs?" "I wonder who's driving." "Will they get into college?" "What chance do they have of getting a job/buying a house/having children…?" As soon as you become a parent, you don't just worry about your own place in society, you worry about your child's, too. And because you can't really control them any more than you can control a car from the back seat, it feels like worrying is all you can do.

Diet

Food should not make us anxious, should it? Unless, that is, you have a tendency to consume poison.

When we eat or drink anything that goes against Mother Nature's guide, our natural survival mechanism finds a way of letting us know. That could be pain in the form of indigestion, constipation, diarrhea, or vomiting… or it could be guilt, disappointment, or feeling that we're not in control.

These emotions trigger chronic anxiety. We worry a lot about not being the perfect shape and weight, and we worry about our addiction to foods that make us fat. Our hunter-gatherer ancestors didn't have these anxieties. Their lifestyle kept them in the perfect shape and weight to hunt and survive.

Today, our obsession with shape and weight is more about appearance. Image consciousness has been heightened by social media, where we post pictures of ourselves and compare ourselves to others, and anything unfavorable becomes a source of misery.

Yet, despite this obsession, we devour junk food that has the opposite effect on our appearance of the one we want.

Health

We are lucky enough to live in an age in which medical science works wonders to keep us alive. Yet there are always new health scares to keep us on edge.

Every ache and pain, every twinge and tweak can send us rushing to the Internet to find out what we might have. "Is it bad, doctor? Am I going to live?" We worry about our own health and

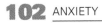

we worry about the health of our loved ones. We share horror stories about freakish ailments and injuries, as if getting closer to the full horror somehow protects us from being affected.

But we are affected. We lie awake and worry about what might be wrong with us. We conjure up catastrophic scenarios. And there are enough miserable health conditions out there to keep us worrying forever more… if that's what we choose to do.

The fact is, with all these anxieties, we have a choice. We do have control. It's just a case of learning how to let go of the anxiety and regain a sense of reality.

Sleep loss

Anxiety causes sleep loss, which is in turn a cause of anxiety. Because sleep is such an important part of our life cycle, we are naturally tuned in to any signs that we are lacking sleep.

If you knew that every night you would be tormented by a demon that made you fretful and miserable, you would spend the whole day feeling anxious about it. Sleep loss has the same effect. When you know something bad is coming, you worry about it.

This is both an instinctive anxiety and an intellectual one. The Incredible Machine needs sleep, and when it doesn't get it, things start to break down and our senses tell us there is a problem. But we also know intellectually that sleep deficiency is bad for us, that it will affect our mood and performance and can make us ill.

So the longer we suffer from insomnia, the more anxious we will become, making it harder to achieve the peace of mind and physical relaxation required for unbroken sleep.

CHOOSING CALM

As with the lifestyle choices we have focused on in previous chapters, we get stuck with anxiety because we don't realize we have a choice. We assume that anxiety is a condition that happens to us in certain circumstances, and that we just have to endure it until those circumstances change.

In the case of sleep loss in particular, it's pretty obvious that the circumstances will not change until the anxiety goes away. The same is true of all the other anxieties we have covered in this chapter. You need to deal with the anxiety first and then the circumstances will change.

So how do you overcome anxiety? First, let us establish how NOT to overcome anxiety. Not with a drink. Not with a cigarette. Not with any sort of drug, or by "comfort" eating. These are the so-called "crutches" we typically turn to when we're feeling anxious. Do they help? On the contrary—they make matters worse.

Not only do drugs and junk food create a physical feeling of unease as we withdraw from the initial fix, the knowledge that we are dependent on these things is an intellectual source of anxiety.

Addictions do not create the right head space for overcoming anxiety. They simply create anxiety.

The way to overcome anxiety is to connect with Mother Nature's guide, pay attention to your senses, and release your grip on your anxieties. You gain control by letting go. It takes practice because anxiety naturally makes you tense. You instinctively tighten your grip. But there is nothing to hold onto because these are perceived threats that haven't become real yet and may never do so.

Anxieties always feel worse at night. That's because we are powerless to do anything about them while we're lying in bed. They just go around and around your brain, avoiding any attempts to resolve them through thought. Problems become much less frightening when you are able to do something active to tackle them.

When you're feeling anxious, ask yourself if the threat is real or perceived. If it is real, take the necessary steps to eradicate it. If it is the middle of the night, resolve to do something about it in the morning. If it is perceived, let it go. Don't keep yourself awake trying to solve problems that don't exist.

By following this simple process of questioning, you will start to figure out which anxieties need attention and which do not. Your level of anxiety will fall and you will begin to reverse the vicious circle.

With all the anxieties covered so far, there is a basis to the projected fear, whether that's money, work, relationships etc. But what if your perceived fears are based on brainwashing? Through the influence of role models and advertising, you can be made fearful of threats that don't exist at all and never will.

It's time to tackle the fear of success.

Chapter 9

TWO FEARS

•*FEAR OF FAILURE* •*FEAR OF SUCCESS*
•*A TUG-OF-WAR* •*REMOVE ALL DOUBTS*

In Chapter 7, we said that there are two myths that lead us into the trap and keep us there:

1. The myth that drinking, smoking, eating junk food, gambling, and burning the candle at both ends gives you pleasure or a crutch.

2. The myth that stopping or changing our behavior, will be hard and leave us feeling miserable.

We have established that the key to overcoming your sleep problem is to change some of your food, drink, drug consumption and lifestyle choices, but somewhere in your mind there might be a sense that this will not be a happy experience.

That's perfectly normal. All our food, drink and drug consumption, and all our lifestyle choices are made in the pursuit of happiness. Nobody chooses to smoke, for example, in order to suffer from the misery of lung cancer, heart disease, emphysema, or any of the other life-shortening diseases associated with smoking, not to mention the vast financial cost, the smell, the loss of taste, control, and the slavery of being a drug addict. Smokers start smoking because they are sold the idea that it's a pleasurable, relaxing, fun, sophisticated, stress-relieving, and enjoyable thing to do. In other words, that it provides some form of pleasure or supportive benefit.

So when it comes to stopping, it's not as simple as replacing cigarettes with some other substitute, like patches or nicotine gum. You need to unravel the brainwashing and remove the first myth: that smoking gives you some kind of pleasure or a crutch.

The same is true of all our sleep-disruptive lifestyle choices and food, drink, or drugs that might be causing us sleep issues—even if we don't feel that we are technically addicted to them. If we are to change them, we must first recognize that they do nothing for us, so that there is no feeling of sacrifice.

In this way we remove the second myth: that changing, amending, or stopping certain food, drink, or drugs will be hard and make us miserable, as will any lifestyle choice changes we attempt. If you believe that your diet or lifestyle choices give you pleasure, benefit, and happiness, then of course you will feel deprived if you deny yourself, and the temptation to go back to them will always nag you. Remember the Big Monster?

With Easyway, you don't have to use willpower to resist the temptation. You remove the temptation altogether.

Let's examine that second myth more closely.

FEAR OF FAILURE

Why do we believe that changing any of our chosen behaviors will be hard? There are two main reasons: first, we may have tried and failed in the past; second, we are constantly told that it's hard.

The world is full of people vowing to quit smoking, cut down on their drinking, eat less etc. Doesn't it strike you as odd that these are all supposed to be pleasures, yet we're always promising to do them less? Say you had a genuine pleasure in life, such as playing tennis. You wouldn't go around telling people you're trying to cut down on the amount of tennis you play. You would want to play as often as you can. It's a clear indication that these so-called pleasures are not what they are made out to be.

So everywhere you look there is someone trying to quit smoking, observe Dry January, cut out carbs etc—and boy do they let us know about it!

Addiction works like a trap. Anyone who has tried and failed to quit will know that it leaves you feeling more firmly trapped than you did before. You've seen movies where a captive is thrown into a room and the door locked behind them. The first thing they do is run to the door and try the handle. This confirms their predicament: they really are locked in. Trying and failing to quit has the same effect on an addict. It reinforces the belief that you are in a trap from which there is no escape.

This can be a crushing experience. Whereas you once might have told yourself you will quit one day, just not yet, now you are faced with the grim realization that you can't kid yourself anymore. Many addicts conclude that the best way to avoid this misery is to avoid trying to quit in the first place. As long as you never try to escape, you will always be able to tell yourself that escape is possible. It is only when you try to escape and fail that you have to admit it's impossible.

This is the twisted logic of addiction, and you can see how self-defeating it is; but there are millions of intelligent people who continue to delude themselves in this way. They prefer to continue suffering from the misery of addiction than risk the misery of failure. What they don't realize is that the door only remains shut if you use the wrong method to open it.

BY PROTECTING YOURSELF FROM THE FEAR OF FAILURE, YOU GUARANTEE THAT YOU WILL FAIL.

It's like wanting to be a tennis champion but protecting yourself from the fear of failure by never playing any matches. Your chances of becoming a tennis champ are zero.

With addiction, the fear of failure is the fear of remaining an addict. But you're already an addict, so you're fearing something that has already happened. If you continue to avoid even trying to escape, you guarantee that you will feel like a failure for the rest of your life.

For people who do succeed in their ambitions, like the tennis champion who does play matches, fear of failure is a positive force. It focuses the mind, drives you to practice harder, and gives you an energy that is compelling. Whether you are an aspiring tennis player or you just want to improve your diet, the same is true for all of us: when channeled positively, the fear of failure can magnify your abilities.

By trying to change some of your food, drink, and drug intake and some of your lifestyle choices, you give yourself a chance of successfully curing your sleep problem. By trying to change them with Easyway, you give yourself the best possible chance. By following all the instructions in order, from beginning to end, you cannot fail.

FEAR OF SUCCESS

Why do we believe that changing any of our sleep-disruptive diet and lifestyle choices will be miserable? Surely it's a wonderful relief to break free from that feeling of being trapped. But because of the twisted way in which addiction works, when you're in the trap, you don't see it like that.

We can all imagine the misery of being sent to prison and find it hard to understand why anyone who has spent time in one would re-offend and run the risk of going back in. But this happens with depressing regularity, particularly among prisoners who have spent a long time behind bars.

It's easy to assume that they re-offend because they haven't learned the error of their ways—but often it's because they actually want to go back inside. They yearn for the "security" of prison. Life on the outside is alien and frightening for them; it doesn't adhere to the same routine or the same guidelines. It's not what they know, and they don't feel equipped to handle it.

When you believe that your diet and lifestyle choices give you some kind of benefit or crutch, the thought of living without them is also frightening. You don't know how you will cope without your usual routine. You think you will have to go through some uncomfortable transition period to break free, and that if you succeed in changing, you will be condemned to a life of sacrifice and deprivation.

In short, you fear that you won't be able to enjoy life anymore.

It is perfectly understandable that this fear should hold anyone back from trying to make diet or lifestyle changes. Who wants to stop enjoying life? But is the fear itself a rational one? Is it a real fear? Or is it an illusion based on brainwashing?

A TUG-OF-WAR

The fear of success is far more powerful than the fear of failure when it comes to changing your diet or lifestyle choices. It is virtually impossible to commit to a decision that you believe is going to make life less enjoyable.

If you've tried to change some of your diet and lifestyle choices in the past in an attempt to solve your sleep issue, it's likely that you did so with a gloomy reluctance that the misery of missing out on certain things might be less severe than the misery of not being able to sleep. Even if you managed to live that way for a while, it's likely that eventually your old diet and lifestyle choices slipped back in, with the sleep problem firing up all over again.

It's like a tug-of-war: at one end is the fear of how to survive feeling tired, lethargic, and exhausted all the time, and at the other end is the fear of how to cope without one's usual diet and lifestyle. It's a tug-of-war of fear—with fear at both ends. Both fears are caused by the same thing: the diet and lifestyle choices that cause our sleep issue. We feel that the only way we stand a chance of breaking free is to make huge sacrifices in diet and lifestyle. It never occurs to us that the elements of those areas that need to change aren't bringing us pleasure or enjoyment or support or benefit. In fact, they're dragging us down. That's why it's so important to understand the difference between real pleasure and the illusion of pleasure.

Fear lies at the root of all addictions and behavioral issues. It is the force that makes the trap so ingenious, because it works in reverse. It plays on the false belief that your worst enemy is your best friend. The thing you rely on to make you feel secure is the very thing that is actually making you feel vulnerable.

When you wake up in the morning feeling exhausted after another night of broken sleep, the Big Monster will tell you that you need a strong cup of coffee. But you know that caffeine is the enemy of sleep.

It's obvious that in order to break the vicious circle you need to stop drinking coffee. There is no need to mope about it. You know that all coffee does for you is ensure that the broken nights continue. It doesn't give you a genuine high. Any feeling of pleasure is just the partial and temporary relief from the craving caused by the caffeine from the previous cup of coffee leaving your system. In fact, it's worse than that. Because the temporary relief from the craving for, and the withdrawal from, caffeine occurs after having the coffee, you do feel better than you did a moment before. This reinforces the belief that the coffee provides a boost.

It's like the feeling you get when you take off a pair of tight shoes at the end of a long day. Would you deliberately wear tight shoes just to get that relief? Would you regard tight shoes as a source of pleasure that you couldn't live without?

Every time you feel that illusory boost the Big Monster grows: your belief in what the coffee does for you, and how awful, exposed, and abandoned you'd feel without it.

As long as you continue to believe that the unhelpful diet and lifestyle choices give you pleasure or a crutch, you will be caught in the tug-of-war of fear and it will make it virtually impossible for you to change. But there is an easy way to win the tug-of-war. Just stop.

Caffeine is a great example. Undoubtedly, if you consume caffeine it is contributing to your sleep issue, creating misery and fear. Because you've been fooled into believing that caffeine does something positive for you, you believe that life will be miserable without it. If you can understand that, in fact, caffeine provides you with absolutely nothing but misery, then any fear of living without it disappears... as does the inclination to consume it.

REMOVE ALL DOUBTS

We are so used to making "action plans," but how about, for once, creating an "inaction plan:" things to consider removing from your schedule, or at least preparing to reduce, reschedule, or change.

Think about your diet and lifestyle choices, and which you might need to address in order to be free of sleep issues. Make a list. You probably know them already, but writing them down, and perhaps adding to them as you read through this book, will help you a) consider whether you need help to make the changes and b) whether you're satisfied that you can make the changes happily, rather than with a feeling of doom and gloom.

Here are some questions that should help you create your list. Please don't be alarmed or afraid of the sheer number of questions and issues raised. Chances are some of them, rather than all of them, are responsible for your sleep issue. Consider this an exciting exploration of your behavior, food, drug, and drink intake and how they might be hindering your attempts to achieve great sleep. Also, please don't be put off by the element of repetition; I want you to read carefully through this text, taking in every single word, relating to every single issue, even if it feels frustrating, pedestrian, and repetitive:

1. Do you drink coffee or energy drinks containing caffeine?

    • Do you understand how using stimulants for prolonged periods of time causes fatigue, rather than relieves it?

    • Do you understand that the consumption of any coffee or caffeine, at any time of day, is likely to be a major factor in your sleep issue?

- Should you be happy or sad that you can decide to change from being a caffeine drinker to a non-caffeine drinker?

- Why not be happy to change, especially since you should find it easy, and not miss it at all? Not only will it feel fabulous, but you will also be maximizing your chances of achieving GREAT SLEEP.

2. Do you eat a diet high in processed and starchy carbohydrates (bread, pizza, pasta, rice, potatoes, salty snacks, etc)?

   - Do you understand that these items manipulate blood-sugar levels, which causes highs and lows in energy levels, fatigue, and mood?

   - Do you understand that consistent blood-sugar levels, rather than the extreme highs and lows caused by the consumption of processed and starchy carbs, aid restful sleep?

   - Should you be happy or sad that you can decide to change from eating a diet high in processed and starchy carbs that causes you harm?

- Why not be happy to change, especially since you should find it easy, and not miss it at all? Not only will it feel fabulous, but you will also be maximizing your chances of achieving GREAT SLEEP.

3. Do you consume refined sugar every day (candy, chocolate, desserts, sweet nut bars, and other sweet snacks, etc)?

    - Do you understand that these items manipulate blood-sugar levels, which causes highs and lows in energy levels, fatigue, and mood?

    - Do you understand that consistent blood-sugar levels, rather than the extreme highs and lows caused by the consumption of refined sugar, aid restful sleep?

    - Should you be happy or sad that you can decide to change from eating a diet containing high levels of refined sugar that causes you harm?

    - Why not be happy to change, especially since you should find it easy, and not miss it at all? Not only will it feel fabulous, but you will also be maximizing your chances of achieving GREAT SLEEP.

4. Do you consume fruit that has been processed and is therefore not in its natural state (this includes fruit juices, smoothies and dried fruit)?

    • Do you understand that these items manipulate blood-sugar levels, which causes highs and lows in energy levels, fatigue, and mood?

    • Do you understand that consistent blood-sugar levels, rather than the extreme highs and lows caused by the consumption of fruit that is not in its natural state, aid restful sleep?

    • Should you be happy or sad that you can decide to change from eating a diet containing high levels of processed fruit that causes you harm?

    • Why not be happy to change, especially since you should find it easy, and not miss it at all? Not only will it feel fabulous, but you will also be maximizing your chances of achieving GREAT SLEEP.

5. Do you eat your evening meal early in the evening, or later? Did you know that eating your evening meal later, rather than earlier in the evening, increases the chances that you will a) gain weight and b) have poor sleep? The situation is even worse if your evening meal contains caffeine, refined

sugar, processed and starchy carbs, fruit that is not in its natural state, and salty or sweet snacks.

- Do you understand that eating later rather than earlier, especially consuming the items above, provides you with energy that you do not require at night, and manipulates blood-sugar levels, which causes highs and lows in energy levels, fatigue, and mood?

- Should you be happy or sad that you can decide to change from eating your evening meal later, and perhaps omitting some of the items you include in those meals, both of which cause you harm?

- Why not be happy to change, especially since you should find it easy, and not miss those items or eating later at all? Not only will it feel fabulous, but you will also be maximizing your chances of achieving GREAT SLEEP.

6. Do you get a reasonable amount of exercise each day? Did you know that daily moderate aerobic exercise increases your chances of sleeping well? It also particularly benefits the deeper areas of sleep, where the brain and body have a chance to rejuvenate. Exercise helps your state of mind and your mood, which also helps with sleep. Far from having to run miles or spend hours pumping iron in the

gym, a couple of 30-minute walks, at a decent pace, can make all the difference.

- Do you understand that if you don't get much exercise, simply incorporating a couple of 30-minute walks into your daily routine can help you sleep and improve your mood?

- Should you be happy or sad that you can decide to change from getting little or no exercise, which causes you tremendous harm and is one of the causes of your sleep issue?

- Why not be happy to change, especially since you should find it easy, enjoyable, and beneficial in many ways. You will not only feel fabulous, you will also be maximizing your chances of achieving GREAT SLEEP.

7. Do you do vigorous exercise mid- or late evening? Regular exercise is essential for mind, body, and sleep, but exercising too late can cause a few issues for some people: a) people often wait until after their evening workout to eat their evening meal, and eating later, rather than earlier, isn't ideal; and b) vigorous exercise causes the body to release endorphins, which can stimulate brain activity and be unhelpful for sleep.

- Do you understand that if you do vigorous exercise in the evening, the earlier you do it the better?

- Should you be happy or sad that you can decide to change from exercising and eating too late in the evening, factors that are perhaps combining to be one of the causes of your sleep issue?

- Why not be happy to change, especially since you should find it easy, enjoyable, and beneficial in many ways. You will not only feel even better than you do at the moment, you'll also be maximizing your chances of achieving GREAT SLEEP.

8. Do you watch TV or stream shows on a phone, tablet, or laptop shortly before you go to bed? Did you know that this can cause serious sleep issues? Of course you did! But have you done anything with that knowledge? Maybe you addressed it for a while, or attempted to, but found that either it made no difference or that it was too difficult, or unsatisfactory to avoid or change permanently. Who wants to avoid watching their favorite shows? No one. Certainly not someone who enjoys chilling out with movies, soaps, dramas, series, documentaries, sports, music videos, etc. Although we do find it relaxing to watch that stuff, the blue light that emanates from devices greatly reduces your chances of a good night's sleep. It tricks our brains

into thinking it's daytime and prevents our body from producing melatonin. Taking melatonin supplements is not the antidote to that issue—changing our behavior is.

The earlier you unplug those devices before bedtime, the better. But if you can do it an hour before bedtime, and/or switch your TV, phone, tablet, or laptop to night mode, or use a physical filter, or even night/blue-light-blocking glasses, all the better.

- Do you understand that turning off your blue-light-emitting devices a while before bedtime and/or using night mode filters, or night/blue-light glasses will not only enhance your bedtime routine but also help you sleep?

- Should you be happy or sad that you can decide to change from not turning off blue-light-emitting devices earlier, and not using red mode/night mode filters, or night/blue-light-blocking glasses—factors that are undoubtedly some of the causes of your sleep issue?

- Why not be happy to change, especially since you should find it easy, enjoyable, and beneficial in many ways. You will not only feel even better than you do at the moment, you'll also be maximizing your chances of achieving GREAT SLEEP.

OK. I'm sure you get the drift. In fact I've probably provided a few more examples than necessary, and perhaps tested your patience. I make no apologies for doing so; I really want you to think again about the way you think about your sleep issue. Get some fresh insights by applying the kind of wording I've used in the examples above to other factors that you can list.

This isn't an exhaustive list by any means, but here are some more issues for you to continue the exercise with:

9. Do you watch TV shows, movies, or engage on social media on a phone, tablet, or laptop in bed? Is it possible to avoid that? Almost certainly. Try to keep your bedroom, and even more importantly your bed, for cherished sleep and intimacy. Retiring to bed for a night's sleep should be a wonderful, relaxing retreat to a special, safe place— neither the bedroom nor the bed should become a place to "hang out" watching TV, gaming, or flitting through social media. Think about it: how can you make your bed and bedroom more special? Recapture it for its true role, a special place for sleep and intimacy (not that intimacy should be necessarily restricted to that arena, of course).

10. Do you scroll through social media shortly before going to bed? Why? Does it feel like a "wind-down" activity most of the time? Probably not. Definitely consider abstaining from social media for a while prior to retiring to bed,

keeping it out of the bedroom and protecting yourself from blue light etc.

11. Do you have a good bedtime routine? Keep reading, keep making notes on your "inaction plan" and only add elements to your routine that are specifically designed for, or compatible with, achieving great sleep.

12. Do you make your bed in the morning, and is your bedroom tidy? That probably sounds like an unusual question and brings back memories of parents pleading with us as children to "clean up that mess!". However, it is important to maintain a clean, tidy, uncluttered and neat bedroom, and have your bed already made nicely to encourage great sleep. Retiring to our bed should be a wonderful, pleasing moment, and a made bed invites us to sleep. A few seconds of care in the morning reap results when it's time to go to bed again.

13. What temperature is your bedroom? Your body temperature naturally drops as you sleep, and most people sleep best in a temperature of <u>no more than</u> 64°F. Make sure the temperature of your bedroom is correct before heading for bed.

14. If you get up in the night to go to the bathroom, do you have soft lighting/a nightlight to avoid bright/normal

lights while doing so? Having to turn on lights to get to the bathroom causes unnecessary disruption to someone who wishes to return to sleep. Be sure to keep the room as softly lit as possible.

15. Do you drink alcohol every evening? We'll talk more about this later, but think about your alcohol consumption. If you drink alcohol every day, ask yourself why, how much, and when? It's a touchy subject for many people, and one we tend to shy away from. But if you feel that perhaps you are drinking a little too much, a little too often (or worse), then please do reach out for help. Aside from that, the notion of a beneficial "nightcap" is a myth. It might sedate you somewhat, and for someone with an alcohol issue, it might temporarily halt the nagging physical withdrawal and the mental craving, but those return very quickly and act as a disruption to getting to sleep, rather than an aid. But in either case—whether you are a "normal drinker" or otherwise—research has proven that just one alcoholic drink can impair and prevent the restorative benefits of sleep, causing you to sleep less restfully and wake up more frequently. The same goes for cannabis.

16. Do you smoke or vape? We'll talk more about this later, but think about it. You might think smoking or vaping keeps you company at night during those periods when you can't sleep, so it's natural to be reluctant to let go of it

for that reason alone—aside from all the other perceived benefits you believe it provides you with. But if you understood that, far from being any kind of comfort or benefit, smoking and vaping not only provide you with neither, but are also a significant cause of your sleep issue, would you at least consider making a change?

At this point let's focus on the sleep impact of smoking and vaping. Smokers take longer to fall asleep, sleep for shorter periods, and spend less time in deep, restorative sleep. That's aside from the respiratory problems that smoking causes, like sleep apnea and asthma. Interestingly, it's worth keeping in mind that secondhand smoke also affects sleep; those who are exposed to smoke in the home are more likely to report poor sleep than those who are not.

Nicotine in any form, including vaping devices, is likely to cause an issue with sleep. Vapers often experience the same sleep issues as smokers and can also suffer from nighttime breathing issues (whether they're daily or non-daily users). Aside from the often unregulated chemicals in vape liquid, nicotine acts in the same inefficient way as caffeine, as a stimulant, and causes issues with your sleep cycle, deep sleep etc.

As a former chain smoker, I fully appreciate the negativity with which you might view the prospect of stopping smoking. I experienced endless periods of misery and torture in my many failed attempts to quit. In fact, it was those experiences that made the ease with which I eventually quit such a revelation. How could something that had been so hard suddenly have become so easy?

Don't panic. You don't have to put this on your list... but at least open your mind to it—especially since there's an easy and pain-free way of breaking free of smoking or vaping.

17. Do you ever do nothing—have a "quiet time," a moment of reflection? Most of us have busy lives with barely a moment to ourselves. Think about how you could incorporate some real downtime/quiet time in the lead-up to bedtime. It only needs to be a matter of minutes. Mindfulness is a great practice, and can help you grow to really appreciate the moment.

18. Do you nap during the day? Whereas a short nap might be useful if you feel so inclined, anything longer than 10 or 20 minutes, especially late in the day, can impact negatively on your quality of sleep.

19. Do you take sleeping pills or supplements to help you sleep? Do they work? If not—why take them? If they do work, why are you reading this book? Depending on what you're taking, if it's not providing you with the solution it promises, you should consider whether there is any point in taking it. We think we can pop a pill and make everything better, but in the vast majority of cases, we're

paying good money for something that's far less effective than obtaining it naturally. Look at all the factors in this long list that can impact negatively on your sleep. We're up to #**19** already! What do you think is more likely to bring you success and help you achieve your objective? Paying through the nose to take an increasing number of pills or supplements, many of which are only suitable for short-term use and are proving to be spectacularly unsuccessful in your search for great sleep? Or make some simple changes in a constructive, cheerful, positive way?

20. Do you have a light-free bedroom (blackout blinds, absence of digital displays etc.)? It's an obvious point, and one you're probably aware of. Have you done anything about it? Are your blackout blinds correctly installed? Do they perform the function they're intended for? If so, that's great. If not, revisit the issue now. It's way easier to introduce helpful light to wake you up beautifully in the morning than it is to ignore unhelpful light when you are trying to achieve and maintain great sleep. The light from digital displays can cause serious problems. Get rid of them or cover them up.

21. Do you find yourself thinking through stressful situations, worries, and anxieties as you prepare for sleep? This is quite common, as is a partner who waits until bedtime to discuss serious or weighty issues. Asking your partner to

be mindful of your winding-down process as part of your new bedtime routine should be enough to dissuade them from doing anything that might interfere with that.

Even if it isn't instigated by a partner, bedtime can be when our worries and stresses invade. Establishing tools and strategies to prevent that from happening is as important as tools and strategies to relieve it when it occurs—especially if the thoughts pop into your mind when you wake up at night and prevent you from getting back to sleep. More about this issue later.

22. What do you do if you feel extremely tired, struggle to keep your eyes open, or nod off in the evening? It can be hugely frustrating to experience this and fight it off only to eventually get to bed and be unable to sleep. Consider an early night. We sometimes worry that we might end up waking up at 4am or 5am if we go to bed early—but is that really a problem if we achieve brilliant, healthy, restorative sleep by then? If you're sleep-deprived, early nights are likely to be a short-lived necessity as your body and brain adjust to you getting that great-quality sleep. But why not try it and see how it goes—especially if you learn to welcome an early morning rather than fear it.

Once you have addressed any diet issues and lifestyle issues, you will experience:
A greater feeling of control

More confidence

Less stress and anxiety

No fear

All of which lead to...

BETTER SLEEP.

A WORD ABOUT SLEEP APNEA

This is a sleep disorder that should not be ignored. It involves a person's breathing repeatedly stopping and starting, often causing the sufferer to wake up with a start or a sudden gasp. If you snore loudly and feel tired even after a full night's sleep, you might have sleep apnea, and should see your doctor; it can cause other health issues if not treated. There are lots of things that can be done, but in the most common types of the condition (obstructive and central sleep apnea) the following symptoms occur:

- Loud snoring (although not everyone with the condition snores)
- Episodes in which you stop breathing during sleep—which could be reported by another person
- Gasping for air during sleep

- Awakening with a dry mouth
- Morning headaches
- Difficulty staying asleep (insomnia)
- Excessive daytime sleepiness (hypersomnia)
- Difficulty paying attention while awake
- Irritability

In the least common type of the condition (central sleep apnea) the sufferer's brain fails to send signals to the breathing muscles, resulting in them making no effort to breathe for a short time, often waking up with shortness of breath and/or experiencing difficulties getting to sleep or staying asleep.

In most cases, there are common factors that increase the risk of sleep apnea, including **being overweight** (fat deposits around the upper airway causing obstruction—or a thicker neck circumference narrowing airways); use of **alcohol, cannabis, sedatives, tranquilizers or opioids** (which relax the throat muscles); **smoking** and **vaping** (inflammation and fluid retention in the upper airway); and nasal congestion.

It's notable that many of these risk factors can be eliminated by making better lifestyle choices and eliminating sleep-disruptive food, drinks, and drugs, as highlighted throughout this book. Implement them and you should reduce your risk considerably; but certainly consult your doctor if you think you might have sleep apnea.

You have every reason to make these new choices and no reason not to. If you could look into the future and see how good you'll feel in a few weeks, you would be amazed. We find it hard to believe that cutting out the things we think make us happy can actually make us happier. And we're brought up to be resistant to change, and are wary of it—even change for the better.

But ask yourself this: are you really enjoying life now, as someone who can't sleep? Isn't the very fact that you are reading this book evidence that all is not well?

You have been tricked into believing that life without certain substances, or making lifestyle changes, is miserable. You're not alone in this. The majority of humanity is subjected to the same brainwashing throughout our lives.

You are aware of the misery associated with smoking, alcohol issues, obesity, gambling, digital addiction etc, but perhaps you regard that misery as the extreme end of the scale and you tell yourself you are nowhere near that.

But here's the indisputable fact: your diet and lifestyle choices are disrupting your sleep.

How serious does it have to get before you make a change?

The only reason you might not see the solution as simple is because you have been brainwashed into the tug-of-war of fear. Once you can see that there is nothing to fear, that you are not giving up anything or depriving yourself in any way, change is easy.

So how many changes would you like to make to rid yourself of your sleep problem?

It's stating the obvious that the more changes you make, the greater your chances of success. It's essential that you get it clear in your mind that these lifestyle choices, as well as problematic food, drink, and drug consumption, do absolutely nothing positive for you whatsoever. Understanding how they fool you into thinking that they do, in fact, do something for you is key.

EASY WINS!

These are easy wins, easy decisions; they probably stand out for you because they seem like such easy changes to make. In the past, you might have attempted to make some or all of these changes and been surprised to find it harder to live with than you expected. This time, though, instead of making the changes in a nervous, reluctant, "beaten before you start" way, you're going to embrace the changes and not only live with them, but thoroughly revel in them, knowing that you are taking the only action required to maximize your chances of achieving great sleep.

MAKE AN EFFORT!

There are items on the list that require you to take some action. There's nothing complicated or even expensive, but you're almost certainly resistant to undertake them simply because it initially requires a little action. Blackout blinds, for example. You might already have them, and they don't work satisfactorily; or you might feel that you can't afford them. If that's the case, a large piece of cardboard (which can be decorated on both sides for aesthetic purposes) cut to the size of your bedroom window can create an excellent, no-cost blackout blind—you just slot it into place at bedtime (and if you're particularly artistic, you can hang it on the wall as art during the day). At the height of summer, when you need to keep the window open for ventilation, perhaps you can resort to a sleep mask. But if you can do without it, you'll avoid the relative encumbrance of wearing one.

Go that extra mile and target as many easy wins from the list as you can.

NOT SO FAST!

Before you move on, I'm going to ask you to take another look at that list and identify the lifestyle, food, drink, and drug choices you're most reluctant to change. You've already added the "easy wins" to your list; now it's time for you to really consider making the changes you're most resistant to even trying. What are they?

They're probably listed below, aren't they?

- Avoid all coffee or energy drinks containing caffeine

- Avoid processed and starchy carbohydrates (bread,

pizza, pasta, rice, potatoes, most salty snacks etc)?

- Avoid refined sugar items (candy, chocolate, desserts, sweet nut bars, and other sweet snacks etc)?

- Avoid fruit juice, fruit smoothies, and dried fruit

- Take a couple of brisk 30-minute walks every day

- Avoid watching TV or other programs on a phone, tablet, or laptop shortly before you go to bed, and/or switch your TV, phone, tablet, or laptop to red mode/ night mode or use a physical filter, or night/blue-light-blocking glasses

- Avoid watching TV or other programs/scrolling through social media on a phone, tablet, or laptop in bed. If you live in a one-room apartment where you don't have access to other rooms, then, if possible, use a chair or beanbag for relaxation, rather than the bed

- If you can, keep your bed and bedroom as a special place designed exclusively for two activities: intimacy and sleep.

- Avoid checking social media shortly before going to bed

- Avoid daily consumption of alcohol

- Avoid sleeping pills and supplements—even melatonin

- Stop smoking or vaping

- Allow yourself to go to bed when you're struggling to keep your eyes open, even if it's early in the evening. It's a sign of serious fatigue—take notice of it.

You don't have to adopt every single one of the above changes, but the more you do adopt, the better your chance of experiencing great sleep.

WARNING!

Can you take it too far? It really is important that you understand the gravity of the likely outcome of adopting too many, or even all, of these changes. You should perhaps brace yourself mentally for what will follow. You will experience some extraordinary, life-changing developments not only in the quality of your sleep, but also a massive increase in energy, mental acuity, happiness, weight loss, improved body shape, enhanced appearance of not only your body but also of your skin and eyes, and a massive, persistent, ongoing boost in your self-esteem and confidence. Who would want that?

Of course, my tongue is firmly in my cheek, and I would encourage you to take this as far as you possibly can. We only have one life. Why spend it feeling constantly downtrodden, tired, lethargic, and out of shape, with what feels like the weight of the world on your shoulders? Isn't it time for you to experience true joy? The more changes you take on board, the greater impact you will have on the length, quality, and enjoyment of your future life.

You understand about the Illusion of Pleasure and how it traps you into believing myths, which in turn undermine your desire to change.

If you have any lingering doubts, we must remove them now. Go back and read Chapters 4 to 6 again if you are unclear on any of the points about the illusions that create the fear that underlies all addictions and behavioral issues.

You need to be fully prepared for the sixth instruction:

Never doubt your decision to change.

You have picked up this book because you want to cure your sleep problem. You have come a long way in the process already, and there is nothing to stop you from going all the way. Always keep in mind the emotions that drove you to pick up this book in the first place, and never let doubt creep into your mind. You have nothing to lose and everything to gain.

Sometimes people say they understand all the instructions, but they still have doubts about the method. It seems too good to be true. Surely there must be some willpower involved somewhere along the line.

Let's be absolutely clear: willpower will NOT give you the power you need. It will only do the opposite. If you don't believe it's possible to solve your problem without willpower, that's simply because you have been brainwashed to think that way.

Earlier in this chapter we made the point that if lifestyle choices or food, drink, and drug consumption like smoking, drinking, gambling, and eating junk food are really a source of happiness, why are so many people always trying to quit? Of course you can't escape that fact, because the people constantly trying to quit make a big song and dance about it. They tell us all about the sacrifices they are making and the mental discipline they are applying. Quite naturally we assume that this is what it takes to quit.

But how many of them succeed in quitting for good? Very few. Why? Because they are using the willpower method.

In the next chapter, we will explain why the willpower method so often results in failure, and why making it easy increases your chances of success.

Chapter 10

WILLPOWER

We have established that in order to cure your sleep problem you need to address some of the lifestyle choices and food, drink, and drug consumption that are proven to be sleep-disruptive. This may not have been what you expected when you first picked up this book.

Most sleep-therapy methods offer tips and techniques designed to help you get to sleep or deal with waking up in the middle of the night. They tend to overlook the fact that you might be doing things during your waking hours that give you next to no chance of getting a good night's sleep.

We've already mentioned some simple sleep tips, and there are more to come later in the book. But unless you apply these tips in conjunction with changes in lifestyle, food, drink, and drug consumption to limit or eradicate elements that are sleep-disruptive, they will be about as effective as a cocktail umbrella in a hurricane.

Most of us believe that changing our lifestyle choices, behavioral issues, and tackling our addictions is hard. Exercise, fitness, dieting, quitting smoking, not drinking ... you probably know dozens of people who have stopped and started, stopped and started, time and time again, and every time they fail they blame one thing: willpower.

Or the lack of it.

In this chapter, we will address this myth and show you that there is nothing to fear in changing your lifestyle choices or escaping behavioral issues or addictions; you don't need to draw on all your willpower and suffer through that terrible experience, that crushing feeling of your willpower giving out. It's actually very easy and will make you feel great from the start.

THE WILLPOWER METHOD

From an early age we are told that we can achieve pretty much anything we want if we try really hard. We are also told that the opposite is true: you don't get anywhere if you don't put in the effort. For the most part, this is true. But not when it comes to addiction.

People who rely on willpower in their efforts to overcome addictions never win the tug-of-war. On one side, their rational brain knows they should change because whatever they're doing is affecting their health or behavior, costing them a fortune, controlling their life, and causing misery. On the other side, the Big Monster makes them panic at the thought of being deprived of something they believe helps them, like a crutch, or provides pleasure.

It's this conflict that makes change hard. Whatever you end up doing, whether you quit forever or relapse, you are guaranteed to remain miserable. When your willpower is holding up, you feel deprived; when it gives out, you feel like a failure.

The willpower method requires you to focus on all the reasons for stopping and hope you can last long enough for the desire to eventually go. But as long as you continue to believe that something gives you pleasure or a crutch, the desire for it will never go.

Easyway helps you remove the desire first. When you remove the desire, quitting is as easy as pushing open a door. But if you've ever come across a door with no handle and pushed on the wrong side, where the hinges are, you'll know how even the simplest of tasks can become hard if you go about it the wrong way. The door might budge a tiny bit, but it won't swing open. It requires a huge amount of effort and determination. Push on the correct side and the door opens without you even having to think about it. That's the difference between the willpower method and Easyway.

It's essential that we do make it easy, because making it hard adds to the problem. Encouraging someone to make a vital lifestyle, behavior or addiction change through the use of willpower is like telling them to open a door by pushing on the hinges.

In reality, there is no physical obstacle for you to move. The closed door standing in your way is purely mental—the Big Monster putting up resistance to change.

You only need willpower if you have a conflict of will. In this case the conflict is between what you really want (the freedom to sleep) and what the Big Monster is telling you that you want (to stay in the trap). Our aim is to resolve that conflict by removing one side of the tug-of-war, so that you have no desire to continue with the diet and lifestyle choices that disrupt your sleep.

THE NO-WILLPOWER METHOD

When we say that Easyway helps people make vital changes without using willpower, we are often met with skepticism. Some people assume it's clever wordplay, or some psychological trick to make them think they are not using willpower when they really are.

Let's be quite clear about this: Easyway does not rely on willpower.

The willpower method is what most so-called experts, such as governments and health organizations, prescribe to help people quit nicotine, alcohol, and other drugs, or to diet, get fit etc. And because it is prescribed by so-called experts, there is widespread acceptance that it is the only way to succeed.

But Easyway has consistently disproven this for more than 35 years. Easyway is not only now clinically proven, but rather than just being based on scientific theories, it has always been based on the real-life experiences of addicts and the first-hand knowledge that willpower does not work. In fact, trying to use willpower makes it harder to change.

HOW WEAK-WILLED ARE YOU?

Whatever the addiction—alcohol, nicotine, other drugs, junk food, gambling, gaming, overspending—when people try and fail to quit with the willpower method, rather than blame the method, they tend to blame themselves. They assume that they are weak-willed.

If you think you are unable to quit because you lack the necessary willpower, then you need to re-read Chapter 4 to understand the nature of the trap you're in.

For those of us who have smoked and drunk alcohol, it's easy to recall how much willpower it took to overcome those first revolting alcoholic drinks or puffs of a cigarette before we became immune to the taste. We force ourselves to carry on in spite of the taste, not because of it. It actually takes willpower to get hooked.

Actually, this is one of the most dastardly tricks of the alcohol industry in recent years: they've removed that initial barrier to entry—the revolting taste. They knew that they could only get a certain number of kids to drink hard liquor, especially cheap hard liquor, if their first reaction to trying it was to spit it out or flinch in revulsion. Over the past 20–30 years, the industry has developed all kinds of carbonated low-alcohol drinks to push teenagers (especially girls) from soft drinks onto alcohol consumption. Eventually, new branding was designed to make these drinks appeal to both sexes; soon there was a dazzling array of "shot" beverages, in gaudy, neon-like colors. And today more mature-looking brands, minus the bright colors, exist to keep those same teens drinking shots as they grow into adulthood. It's just cheap, sickly-sweet, sugar-based booze. Depending on your age, you might even have been one of the industry's earliest victims.

We apply willpower to ignore the warnings about addiction,

whether it's to cigarettes, vaping, alcohol, or other drugs; there is plenty of evidence to suggest that addicts are actually very strong-willed, not weak-willed.

It takes a strong will to persist in doing something that goes against all your instincts. Addicts go to great lengths to make sure they can get their fix, and the more severe the addiction, the stronger the will. So-called problem drinkers will organize their daily lives so they can sneak out and buy booze and discreetly consume it at inappropriate times (in the daytime, at work, etc) without arousing suspicion. Smokers will get up early in the morning to make sure they can get their first cigarette before anyone else is up to make them feel ashamed.

Gamblers will borrow money from friends and family but lie to them about what they need it for. All addicts will sacrifice the pastimes they used to enjoy because their only interest in life is satisfying the Little Monster. These are all lifestyle changes forced on people by the power of addiction and it takes a strong will to keep them up.

The world is full of strong-willed people with addictions. Politicians, professional athletes, actors and actresses, singers, writers, business tycoons... the rehab clinics are full of people who have found stellar success and made a name for themselves in such fields. You don't get to the top of any industry if you're weak-willed. It takes determination, persistence, sacrifice, and hard work. So why would someone with the willpower to be a huge success in their field lack the willpower to quit drinking or smoking or eating junk food? The answer is obvious:

WILLPOWER IS NOT
THE WAY TO QUIT.

How did you react when we first mentioned that you would have to change some of your lifestyle choices in order to cure your sleep problem? Did you feel resistance? Wouldn't you describe that as willful?

In fact, it tends to be the strongest-willed people who find it hardest to quit by using the willpower method, because when the door fails to open they won't give up and try to find an easier method; they will force themselves to keep pushing on the hinges until they can push no more.

MULTIPLE ADDICTIONS

Many drinkers are also smokers, gamblers, and overeaters. You might interpret this as further evidence of a weak will—someone who just can't resist temptation. But temptation is the desire to do something you really enjoy. Smokers don't enjoy smoking; it makes them miserable. The same is true of all addicts. They wish they could stop, but they can't. The force that keeps them hooked is not temptation, it's addiction.

There is a connection between multiple addictions, but it is not that they are evidence of a lack of willpower. On the contrary, they are more likely signs of a strong will. What they all share is that they are traps created by brainwashing. And one of the biggest myths is that quitting requires willpower.

It forces us down a road we don't want to take, embarking on a journey we assume we won't enjoy and for which there is no point of arrival.

FOCUS ON DESIRE, NOT DETERMINATION

In this book I'm applying the principles of Easyway, not just to any addictions or behavioral issues that might be impacting negatively on your sleep, but also to the approach you can take to changing everything on your personal list. Rather than starting off with a feeling of doom and gloom, of holding on like a white-knuckle ride, wondering how long you'll last before you fall and your resolve, determination, and desire to change crumble around you, you can start off with a spring in your step, a sense of being set free, of being released, from an unpleasant, uncomfortable, dark dungeon into bright sunshine and glorious fresh air. You won't be missing out on anything after today—you'll be getting rid of a disease.

Not everyone reading this book necessarily has any addictions to resolve, but some will, which is why I'm obliged to cover them in some detail. But please don't make the mistake of believing that just because you're not addicted to anything, this information doesn't relate to you. It certainly does. If nothing else, it will guide and inform your approach to your own freedom, achieving great sleep.

Perhaps you're someone who drinks alcohol but doesn't think they have an issue with it. That's great; you'll have absolutely no problem cutting out alcohol. If, however, you have an inkling, or indeed are already fully aware that you do have an issue with alcohol, and you've tried and failed in the past to stop, please be reassured—you will break free. See how it goes after reading this book. If you struggle to quit booze, then you can by all means address as many other items on your list as you can… and still succeed. At that time, or before, you may wish to address the alcohol issue itself, in which case, please contact us for free advice and guidance. My alcohol book costs less than a bottle of cheap gin, and our live group seminars come with a money-back guarantee and are now also available online.

The same principle applies to all the addiction issues we've highlighted. If you take on board what you've read already, if you keep reading while following all the instructions, then you will succeed in resolving your sleep issue. If, in spite of that, you fail to quit one or some of the addiction issues, or behavior or diet issues, then we are here to help—whether it is smoking, vaping, sugar, cocaine, cannabis, or any other issue.

In the meantime, you arrive at your goal as soon as you remove the desire to persist with your lifestyle choice, behavioral or diet issue. You remove the desire by understanding that it does nothing for you whatsoever, and that there is nothing to fear about life without it.

By now you should be pretty clear on both of these points. As long as you believe that you are making a sacrifice, you will never reach the end of the road.

The willpower method doesn't only make it harder to quit, it actually encourages you to stay hooked, for two reasons:

1. It reinforces the myth that quitting or achieving change is

hard and, therefore, adds to your fear of failure.

2. It reinforces the myth that life without your little crutch will be joyless, thereby adding to your fear of success.

And in order to alleviate your fears, you revert to the one thing that brought them about in the first place. Thus you become more firmly trapped than before.

Failing to quit with the willpower method makes it harder to try again because failure reinforces the belief that it is impossible to cure your problem. Some people who fail with the willpower method say they feel an enormous sense of relief when they first fall back into the trap, but that it doesn't make them happy. In fact, it makes them even more miserable. Anyone who tells you it's a pleasure is confusing pleasure with the relief of ending their pain. No one thinks, "Great! I've fallen back into addiction." It's not a pleasure; it's a deeply upsetting experience, full of guilt, fear, and hopelessness.

NOTHING TO GIVE UP

The testimony of other quitters who use the willpower method can be damaging to your own desire to quit. There are two types: the Braggers and the Whiners. They either brag about the sacrifices they are making or they whine about them. Either way, they reinforce the myth that quitting demands sacrifice.

Seventh instruction:

IGNORE ANY ADVICE THAT CONFLICTS WITH EASYWAY.

That includes the advice of anyone who claims to have quit by the willpower method. Contrary to what they may tell you, there is no sacrifice. Right now, just by following the instructions in this book, you are making steady progress toward positive, healthy lifestyle choices without any need for willpower.

It should now be clear in your mind that you are not being required to "give up" anything. Nicotine, alcohol, and other drugs do nothing for you whatsoever. Junk food does nothing for you. You only ever thought they did because addiction creates the Illusion of Pleasure. That "pleasure" is nothing more than relief from the craving, which was caused by the drug in the first place.

In your rational mind, you know that these drugs, whether they are stimulants or sedatives, disrupt your sleep, in addition to which they create guilt, self-loathing, helplessness, fear, and other negative emotions that cause anxiety and stress, thus compounding your sleep disruption.

When you understand the way addiction works, you lose the fear of success. Take away the fear and you win the tug-of-war. It's easy.

NO NEED TO WAIT

People who use the willpower method are forever waiting for the moment when the hardship ends and life becomes relaxed and free from the feeling of slavery. But with Easyway there is nothing to wait for. You become happy and relaxed the moment you remove the desire for the drug or behavior.

The fourth instruction was to begin your attempt to change not with a feeling of doom and gloom, but with a feeling of elation. This is the most important decision of your life. By changing your lifestyle choices, you are choosing a life of health and happiness over one of fatigue and misery.

If you have followed all the instructions and understood everything you have read so far, you should be feeling that sense of impending elation and an eagerness to finish the job. You have taken a major step toward freeing yourself from slavery to harmful lifestyle choices and behaviors. You can start living your life again, in control and free.

If you still have doubts, you have either missed something—in which case you need to go back and re-read anything you are stuck on—or there is one last piece of brainwashing that is preventing you from feeling the sense of impending elation. Don't worry. Keep on reading; I have only good news for you.

Some people who try and fail to stop with the willpower method do not put it down to being weak-willed. Instead, they put their failure down to another aspect of their personality over which they have no control. When all other explanations fail them, there is one theory that conveniently provides the excuse they need to stay in the trap: the so-called "addictive personality" theory.

Chapter 11

IS IT SOMETHING ABOUT YOU?

•*WHY ME?* •*THE SCIENTIFIC EXCUSE* •*BIG MONSTER OR PERSONALITY?* •*FILLING A VOID* •*THE LOGICAL ARGUMENT* •*KNOW YOUR ENEMY* •*EMBRACE THE TRUTH*

WHY ME?

The way we respond to insomnia says a lot about our lack of appreciation for the importance of sleep. If you have toothache, you go to the dentist. If you are struggling to see, you book an appointment with the optician. If you have a persistent backache or a suspicious pain anywhere in your body, you visit the doctor.

Yet when we suffer from insomnia, we labor along with it and accept it as a consequence of life. Well, here's news for you: insomnia is not normal. Nor is it inevitable. If you constantly feel tired, it's a sign that there is something wrong—something more critical than a toothache, short-sightedness, or even back pain.

For the reasons we have examined in the preceding chapters, we are reluctant to make the lifestyle changes that will help us sleep because we think that will mean giving up the things we enjoy in life. As you should now understand, this is not the case.

But there is a further reason why we take a different attitude to sleep disruption than to any other ailment. While we react to aches and pains and other ailments as problems we pick up somehow, we tend to regard insomnia as a problem from within—a fault of our own.

"Why me? Because I'm made that way."

The same thinking applies to sleep-disruptive food, drinks, drugs, and lifestyle choices.

"Why can't I quit smoking? Because I have an addictive personality."

"Why can't I lay off the booze? Because I have an addictive personality."

"Why can't I resist chocolate and candy? Because I have an addictive personality."

We wear the label "Addictive Personality" with a strange kind of pride, as if it makes us more interesting somehow. Let's get two things straight:

1. Being an addict is not interesting. It's the opposite of interesting.

2. There is no such thing as an "Addictive Personality." There is only addiction.

In order to cure your sleep problem, it is essential that you dismiss any notion that there might be something in your personality or genetic makeup that condemns you to keep pursuing a sleep-disruptive lifestyle, consuming sleep-disruptive substances, and suffering from insomnia.

THE SCIENTIFIC EXCUSE

Scientists don't help. They always seem to be searching for proof that our behavior is beyond our control. Despite compelling evidence that events which occur in our early years have a strong influence on the way we behave as adults, there is a determination to find a genetic link to everything from happiness to homicide.

You don't need a scientist to tell you that both nature and nurture play a part in who we turn out to be and how we behave—that is abundantly clear. It is also proven that our behavioral tendencies can be altered at any stage in life. In short, your personality was not fixed at birth, nor prior to birth.

The Addictive Personality theory is a godsend for hopeless addicts who refuse to open their minds to the possibility that there is an easy cure. All the other excuses we make so that we can keep drinking or smoking or eating junk food are weak, and we know it—we feel pathetic hearing ourselves say them— but the Addictive Personality excuse is different. It has science behind it! We can say it with gravitas and truly believe what we're saying.

The thinking goes like this: some people have a flaw in their genetic makeup that makes them more susceptible than most to becoming addicted. So, despite their best efforts, they are bound to become addicted and stay addicted.

Let's say for a moment that there really were people born with addictive personalities. What would happen if they were kept from birth on an island with no addictive drugs or activities available to them? Would they behave like addicts? Of course they wouldn't, because you can't become an addict until you take or do something addictive.

The theory gives addicts an excuse to avoid their fear of success by not even trying to quit, and it allows them to go on making the same excuse as they slide deeper and deeper into the trap.

Believing in the Addictive Personality theory does not solve your problem, it merely justifies it.

Do you want to believe that you were born with a genetic predisposition to self-destruction? Did you believe that before you started on your sleep-disruptive lifestyle choices? The fact that you picked up this book suggests that you believe you can be cured. So where does that leave the Addictive Personality theory?

A few so-called "experts" have used the term "Addictive Personality" so often that it is easy to be fooled into believing it is an established condition. It is not. It is a theory and nothing more, largely based on the number of people who have multiple addictions, e.g. drinkers who are also smokers or gamblers, or heroin addicts who smoke and are heavily in debt.

Smoking, drinking, gambling, overeating, debt—they do seem to coincide in a lot of people, don't they? If that is not because they lack willpower, as we stated in the last chapter, could it be because they are more prone to addiction than most people?

That's the theory. But look at the facts. A common approach to quitting, widely recommended by the medical profession, is to substitute one addiction with another. The thinking is that it helps overcome the craving long enough for any desire for the original drug to pass. In reality, it just turns one addiction into two, three, or four. The so-called experts are actively encouraging people to become multiple addicts.

Please get it clear in your mind: all addictions are caused by the same process, but it has nothing to do with your personality or genes. Anyone can avoid addiction, and anyone can break free of addiction too.

BIG MONSTER OR PERSONALITY?

Addiction is a lonely condition, despite the fact that it affects millions of people. Addicts become very insular and convince themselves that they are suffering with a problem that is unique to them. That is why talking to other addicts is so beneficial: it makes you realize that they are experiencing, or have experienced, exactly what you are going through, and you begin to see that addiction is not a weakness in you as an individual but a weakness in the society that brainwashes individuals into the trap.

Just like the belief that you lack the willpower to quit, the Addictive Personality theory is reinforced by failed attempts. If you put all your effort into something but still fail, it is natural to assume that it is beyond your power to solve. Similarly, the Braggers and Whiners who claim to have quit with the willpower method add weight to the theory. They can go months or even years without their fix, but still crave it. That cannot be the effect of the drug in their system—it must be their personality, right?

Wrong. Nobody craves alcohol before they start drinking. Nobody craves a cigarette before they start smoking. The craving has nothing to do with their personality; it is the Big Monster, which was created when they started on the drug and which they have failed to destroy in their attempt to quit.

Remember, the Little Monster is the very mild, slightly restless feeling you get when you're withdrawing from a drug; the Big Monster is the belief that the fix gives you some sort of pleasure or crutch, and that creates a mental craving, and that the only way to relieve the restless feeling or craving is to take more of the drug. The Big Monster is not the same as your personality. You can destroy the Big Monster and your personality will be better off for it.

The willpower method focuses only on killing the Little Monster. It ignores the Big Monster. Easyway handles both the Little and Big Monsters.

It is not just the Little Monster that can arouse the Big Monster. All sorts of things can create a restless feeling that triggers it: a trauma, a social occasion, hunger, a smell, a picture. As long as you allow the Big Monster to remain alive in your head, you will always be vulnerable to a feeling of deprivation and a craving for forbidden fruit. Braggers and Whiners kill off the Little Monster within days of quitting, but they never kill the Big Monster. That's why, years after quitting, they can still fall back into the trap at a moment's temptation.

The so-called Addictive Personality is nothing more than the Big Monster at large.

Killing the Big Monster is easy, provided you keep an open mind. If you cling to the excuse that you have an Addictive Personality, it means that your mind is not open, and you risk sentencing yourself to a lifetime of slavery.

FILLING A VOID

A question we are often asked is this: if addiction has nothing to do with individual personality, why do some people fall deeper into the trap than others? Why can one person have the occasional drink while another downs the whole bottle and opens another? Doesn't that suggest that one has a personality that's more prone to addiction than the other?

It does point to a difference between them, yes, but the difference lies in their life experience, not in their genetic makeup. We are conditioned by all sorts of variable influences: parental guidance, peer pressure, education, income, opportunity… When we are born, we acquire a sense of emptiness and insecurity, which we spend our lives trying to fill. First, we turn to our mother, then our wider family, then friends, role models, lovers, children, ambitions, hobbies, and so on. At Easyway, we call this the Void.

For some people the void is greater than for others because of their upbringing, the environment in which they live and a whole host of other factors. Such factors will determine how easily they are drawn to harmful lifestyle choices and to what extent they indulge.

The restrictions in our lives also control our behavior. Money and time, for example, restrict the amount you are able to drink or smoke or eat. But if all the restrictions were taken out of the way, we would all tend to consume more, not less, because that's how addiction works.

Look at the people who fall deepest into the trap and you'll find they are the ones with the greatest opportunity, the most money, and the greatest desire because of the way they have been conditioned. You may regard them as hopeless cases. Easyway has seen countless such "hopeless cases" released from the trap simply by reversing the conditioning, unraveling the brainwashing and helping them realize that their little crutch is actually no such thing—it is their mortal enemy.

You may also have noticed that people who don't fall into the trap at all—those lucky ones who can happily say "no"—seem to be a different breed. They make you feel slightly uncomfortable, don't they? You feel much more at home with your fellow addicts, and you appear to share similar character traits.

You might take this to mean that there's a shared personality trait that makes addicts more comfortable in the company of other addicts. But what are those traits? An unstable temperament, which swings between exuberance and misery; a tendency toward excess; a high susceptibility to stress; evasiveness; anxiety; insecurity? These traits are all caused by addiction; they are not the reason you do it.

Addicts feel more comfortable in the company of other addicts for one simple reason: they won't challenge you or make you think twice about your addiction, because they're in the same boat. All addicts know that they're doing something stupid and self-destructive. If you're surrounded by other people doing the same thing, you don't feel quite so foolish.

One of the best things about breaking free from addiction is that you also get freedom from the harmful effect it has on your character. You'll be able to enjoy the company of all sorts of people, addicts, and non-addicts, and you'll probably find that non-addicts stay interesting for longer.

You just need to understand that you didn't become hooked on your lifestyle choices, behaviors, and substances because you have an Addictive Personality. If you think you do, it's simply because you got addicted. This is the trick that addiction plays on you. It makes you feel dependent and believe that there is some weakness in your character or genetic makeup. It distorts your perceptions and thus maintains its grip on you.

THE LOGICAL ARGUMENT

Let's say there is an addictive personality gene. It would be fair to assume that this gene would have appeared in a fairly constant percentage of the world population and in the same geographical concentrations throughout history, would it not? Yet this is not the case.

Smoking statistics, for example, paint a very different picture: in the 1940s more than 80 percent of the UK adult male population was hooked on nicotine; today it's fewer than 25 percent. A similar trend is evident throughout most of Western Europe and North America. So are we to conclude that the proportion of people with addictive personalities has fallen by a whopping 55 percent in just 75 years?

At the same time, the number of smokers in Asia

has soared. Can it really be possible that a genetic trait can rise and fall so rapidly within a few decades, and even transfer itself wholesale from one continent to another?

The statistics make a mockery of the Addictive Personality theory.

KNOW YOUR ENEMY

When you come to change your sleep-disruptive lifestyle choices, you engage in a battle against two monsters. Your chances of winning that battle are greatly improved simply by knowing the two monsters exist and understanding how they work.

Whether the issue on your list has to do with consumption, behavior, or lifestyle choice, we can often view it through the prism of addiction.

Here are some examples to help you do that easily.

- Alcohol, nicotine, cocaine, cannabis, caffeine, and other stimulants and sedatives all interfere with sleep and are clearly all drugs, so it's easy for you to relate to them as a "fix."

- Refined sugar and processed or starchy carbohydrates work in a similarly addictive way by manipulating blood-sugar levels, which in turn interferes with hunger, mood, wellbeing, and energy levels, and therefore disrupts sleep. With that in mind, I'm sure you can relate to their consumption as a "fix" too.

Certain behavioral issues, though, are simply practical issues to consider; therefore we don't need to view them as we might do addictions. But a similar principle applies: we establish the behavior based on false information—the mistaken belief that it is positive behavior.

For example, keeping your bedroom at what you consider to be a lovely, warm temperature, whereas perfect sleep conditions are much cooler than that: no more than 64°F. If you view making a change in temperature as a negative change, you'll be miserable. But get this clearly in your mind: nothing bad is going to happen, and it's exactly the right step for you to take to maximize your chances of great sleep. It might take a little getting used to, but in no time at all it will feel perfectly normal. These are the behavioral changes that you can adopt with a smile on your face.

As soon as you identify a behavior, or in some cases a lack of behavior, as a likely contributor to your sleep issue, you can address it with pleasure rather than a feeling of sacrifice.

What other examples might I use? Eating late in the evening rather than earlier; it's not necessarily something we think about too deeply. But would it be so difficult to adjust that behavior? Should it make us unhappy to do so? Of course not. Likewise, perhaps we should consider eating a lighter meal in the evening than we might during the day. Even if that's a little inconvenient, isn't it worth the effort? The rewards are huge in terms of your quality of sleep.

Not getting enough exercise is something you've probably been planning to address for a while. It seems nicer to collapse in a heap on the sofa at every opportunity—but how does it really make us feel? Not content, and certainly not as content as you might feel after a brisk 30-minute walk before settling down to watch TV.

All these behavioral issues can be viewed in the same way. Think again about them, and about how easy, enjoyable, and life-enhancing they will be to address. Look forward to those changes in behavior, especially those related to TV, social media, smartphone, tablet, or laptop engagement: where, when etc.

Back to those fixes: food, drink, and drugs.

The Little Monster is created with the very first fix. A short while after the drug is used, it begins to leave the body—something that is described as withdrawal. As it withdraws it creates a mild, slightly empty, insecure feeling. It's so slight, it's almost imperceptible.

That feeling didn't exist before you took the drug.

The drug withdrawing from your body created it.

People who never, ever take that drug never, ever experience that feeling.

You take another hit of the drug and that mild, slightly empty, insecure feeling is temporarily relieved. You do feel better than you did a moment before—but remember, it's just the temporary relief of the empty, insecure feeling that was created by the first hit of the drug.

In other words, when you use the drug again, the feeling of relief you experience is simply the ending of the dissatisfied condition that was created by the first hit of the drug. In other words, you take the drug in order to feel like someone who's never taken it.

As addicts, we're soon convinced that each hit of the drug we take relieves the empty, insecure feeling. We simply forget that it was created by the first hit of the drug, and it never occurs to us that each "fix" simply ensures that we'll suffer the withdrawal again. And again. And again.

That, in its simplest form, is how we become convinced that these drugs help us, rather than hinder us.

Even with drugs that we believe create a significant high—is there really one? There's no doubt that a change occurs, but how do we come to define it as pleasurable? If a young child, with no knowledge of cocaine, were given some, they'd experience tremendous distress. They haven't yet been brainwashed into believing in the high. Of course, in the case of sugar, blood-sugar levels are manipulated; this is also referred to as a boost, or a high.

We visualize it as a high, but it really is just "different." With stimulants, of course, we might initially experience a slight boost in energy, but these stimulants simply don't work when used constantly. In fact, they sentence us to a lifetime of tiredness, fatigue, and sleep issues.

How does eating refined sugar (candy, cookies, chocolate, desserts, cakes, pastries etc) and processed/starchy carbs (pasta, rice, potatoes etc) generally make us feel? Fit as a fiddle? Bursting with energy? Full of life? Of course not. Invariably they leave us feeling bloated, heavy, guilty, tired and, in spite of the often large amounts of them we eat, hungry for more. The more you consume, the more tired, lethargic, out of shape, miserable, and guilty you feel. But that Little Monster remains inside us, prompting us to have a just a little bit more of what we think we need.

With regard to drugs or sugar, the Little Monster feeds on each new fix, and when you don't give it what it wants, it begins to complain. This feeling is barely perceptible, like a slight itch, but it is enough to arouse the Big Monster.

This Big Monster is not physical, but psychological. It is created by all the brainwashing that has led you to believe that the fix gives you pleasure, or a crutch, and it interprets the Little Monster's complaints as "I need a fix." Trying to please the Big Monster means trying to satisfy a craving by doing the very thing that caused the craving in the first place.

Every time you get a fix, it temporarily tranquilizes the Little Monster, creating the illusion that the fix has made you relaxed and happy. In fact, all it has done is take you from feeling miserable and restless to feeling OK. Now you will need it again and again just to keep you feeling OK.

But actually you never quite get back to where you were before you started. Look again at the diagram in Chapter 4. Every time you give your body a stimulant, it develops a tolerance against it. So every time you get a fix, you need a bigger dose to get the same boost, and every time it wears off, you sink lower. The longer you go on trying to satisfy the Little Monster, the lower you sink and the more dependent you feel on the stimulant. It makes the Big Monster increase the mental craving.

While the Little Monster is barely perceptible, the Big Monster really can make you miserable. When it is awakened, it fills your head with a sense of deprivation, a frustrated feeling that something is missing, reminding you of all the misinformation you've been given about these choices being a source of pleasure, and compelling you to find another fix. The only "pleasure" you get is the mild relief from the withdrawal symptoms and the tranquilizing of the Big Monster. It's like wearing tight shoes just for the pleasure of taking them off—it's the Illusion of Pleasure and relief.

"Does it really matter if it's just an illusion, as long as it makes me feel better for a moment?"

Imagine that a friend gave you $100. In doing so they told you they'd had a bit of good fortune and wanted to share it with you. It would feel awkward and maybe a little weird, but terribly generous. They seem so kind and happy with their good fortune, so you to accept it with gratitude.

A week or two passes and the friend does the same thing. They give you $100. Another month passes and they do it again. Each time it's easier for you to accept the gift, less awkward, and you stop questioning the whys and the wherefores.

Then, after a few months and countless cash gifts, you discover that you have hundreds and hundreds of dollars missing from your bank account. You check your statements and it becomes clear that your so-called friend has been using your debit card to withdraw money from your account. Each time they took $200 coincides with the date on which they gave you $100. They were actually giving you your own money!

Would you remain grateful to that friend? After all, $100 is $100, isn't it? It is real, isn't it?

Of course not—you'd be devastated at the betrayal and the theft of your money, angry at yourself for being fooled, and angry with the friend for conning you.

How can you view someone giving you $100 as being anything other than kind and generous? It's only when you have all the information, only when you find out that the $100 was already yours and, more than that, the thief has kept $100 for themselves each time, that you see the "gift," and the so-called friend, as they really are. A sham. A con. A rip-off!

If you're thinking, Well, at least they gave $100 of the $200 back to me—they could have taken it all, wake up! Not content with stealing from you, they made a fool of you as well.

In the case of drug and food fixes—they've been conning you for years.

The illusion of pleasure and relief is valueless—and it does matter that it isn't real.

EMBRACE THE TRUTH

Any difficulty you experience in changing the lifestyle choices, behaviors, and habits that disrupt your sleep has nothing to do with your personality and everything to do with the brainwashing you've been subjected to from birth. If you experience cravings for, say, alcohol or junk food or cigarettes, this is a symptom of addiction and is nothing more than a desire to feel the way a non-addict feels all the time.

The thought of "giving up" these choices is frightening if you believe that they give you pleasure or a crutch. When you can see that there is no genuine pleasure or crutch and, therefore, you are not sacrificing anything, this fear disappears.

The hopelessness of the addiction trap makes addicts try to blot out the problem and pretend it doesn't exist. They lie to themselves about the state they're in and laugh it off with other addicts, but deep down they know it's no laughing matter; it's a miserable situation, and if they could end it with a wave of a magic wand they would not hesitate.

Using any excuse just so you can continue pursuing sleep-disruptive behaviors means consigning yourself to a lifetime of fatigue and the risk of serious health problems. Release yourself from the prison. Take your head out of the sand and see things as they really are. There is a wonderful life awaiting you, free from addiction and slavery. You don't need a magic wand; you have something in your hands that is just as effective when it comes to curing addiction and behavioral issues: Easyway. All you have to do is follow the instructions.

Let's recap the instructions so far.

1. Follow all the instructions

2. Keep an open mind

3. Reject anything that goes against Mother Nature's guide

4. Begin with a feeling of elation

5. Question everything you think you know about sleep, addiction, and behavior

6. Never doubt your decision to change

7. Ignore any advice that conflicts with Easyway

If you have followed all the instructions in order, then you have already taken a big step toward solving your problem. You have overcome denial and accepted that you need to make some new choices. You have also taken action to do something about the problem. That is another big step. Now all you have to do is kill the Big Monster, which might undermine your plans. Once the Big Monster is dead, you will find it easy to cut off the supply to the Little Monster, and it will die very quickly.

Remember that this relates to the intake of substances (the addictive element of food, drink and drugs) and the false sense of comfort that sleep-disruptive behaviors seem to provide—all of which combined = the Little Monster.

Remember also that the brainwashing which makes you believe that changing your intake of substances or your sleep-disruptive behavior is hard, that it won't last, and that it probably won't help your situation anyway = the Big Monster.

It's the Big Monster that will try to nag away at your decisions, make you believe you're missing out on something, and tease you to go back to your old substances and behaviors, which you know to be sleep disruptive.

Remember, people who try to make these changes with the willpower method never kill the Big Monster. They think it is enough just to kill the Little Monster.

You have already begun to kill the Big Monster simply by questioning everything you thought was true, and you understand that the way to finish it off is to have a clear understanding of the Illusion of Pleasure and relief.

At this stage, a lot of people say they understand everything completely and are in a hurry to get to the end. But it often turns out that they still retain some belief in the Illusion of Pleasure and relief. As long as you remain fooled by the illusion, you will always be susceptible to feeling deprived.

It's essential, therefore, that we make sure you remove the Illusion of Pleasure and relief completely, and get you to start to trust your instincts.

Chapter 12

SEEING THINGS AS THEY REALLY ARE

•POPULAR MYTHS •WIN THE TUG-OF-WAR
•TRUST YOUR SENSES

POPULAR MYTHS

In order to cure insomnia, you need to create the ideal conditions for a good night's sleep. That includes where you sleep and when you sleep, but also the way you treat your mind and body while you are awake.

Modern life throws up numerous conditions that are disruptive to sleep. We make lifestyle choices that cause stress and anxiety. Whereas we choose to try our first experimental cigarette, I'm sure that you understand already that after that choice doesn't come into it—we become addicted. Sometimes genuine lifestyle choices don't feel like choices at all, like working long hours or worrying about our children.

In Chapter 2, we identified some of the most common sleep-disruptive lifestyle choices, diet, and behavioral issues and showed how they are often interlinked. For example, the effect of drugs like nicotine and alcohol is to increase stress and anxiety, as well as impeding the chemical processes that enable you to sleep.

Stress and anxiety are themselves major sleep disruptors, but many of the aspects of life over which we get stressed and anxious are not genuine threats at all; they are perceived or imaginary threats.

We perceive these threats and we make bad lifestyle choices because we are fed false information from a wide range of influential sources. In short, we are brainwashed. We are very susceptible to brainwashing because we trust human intellect over human instinct. For the most part, we go along with the crowd unquestioningly.

Even when our lifestyle choices begin to backfire, we don't question the information that led us to make those choices; we question our own mental strength and genetic makeup. "What's wrong with me? Why can't I handle this?" When you sum it all up like this, the outlook appears to be pretty bleak for humankind. The aim here is not to paint a picture of doom and gloom, but to capture in a nutshell the nature of the problem so you can understand it quite simply and very clearly.

The problem is as simple as figuring out which side to push on a door with no handles in order to make it swing open.

Because of the brainwashing and the way addiction makes us see things backwards, we spend a lot of time pushing on the wrong side of the door. As you continue to read through this book, the correct side of the door will become obvious, and you will grow increasingly excited about your ability to open it.

You will see that an easy solution to your sleep problem is within your reach. You cannot be held back by a lack of willpower, nor by any aspect of your personality or genetic makeup over which you have no control. Your eyes will be opened to a whole new reality that looks wonderful and helps you make good lifestyle, behavior, and diet choices that lead to genuine happiness.

You will see things as they really are.

But I don't smoke or drink

We have talked a lot about nicotine and alcohol, and used these very common examples of how addiction works and twists our sense of reality. If you neither smoke nor drink, hopefully you have understood the principle and applied it to your own sleep-disruptive lifestyle choices, be they diet, use of devices, gambling, overspending, overworking, late nights, or anything else that has a harmful impact on sleep.

You might be a gambler without realizing it. When you think of gambling, you normally think about wagering money on the horses, or at a casino or, these days, on one of the many online-gambling platforms that are trapping millions of people into addiction.

But gambling goes far beyond these so-called leisure pursuits. Many professions require you to gamble. Should you invest in that machine? Should you do that deal? Should you bid for that piece of work? So many business decisions carry risk, and that risk triggers the fight-or-flight response. Spend too much time worrying about the risks you're taking, and you'll lose sleep. In fact, it's the expression we use: "Don't lose sleep over it." It can come down to something as basic as saying what you think to your boss. Will they appreciate your honesty? Or will they show you the door?

If you regularly feel anxious about the decisions you have to make at work, you need to rethink your appetite for risk and ask yourself if it is worth it. For all that you might gain financially, you might lose in terms of your wellbeing. On the other hand, maybe you just need to become comfortable with risk.

If you find the risk element of your job exciting and compelling, it could be that you have become addicted to it and are not aware of the harm it is doing to you. If you have a sleep problem and risk plays a regular role in your work, there is the place to start looking for your solution. Again, rather than be excited by risk, become comfortable with it.

The brainwashing and the trap work in the same way for any harmful lifestyle choice. It's important that you examine all your lifestyle choices and ask, "Is this making me happy, or is it harming me?" Your lifestyle choices need to create the ideal conditions for sleep. If any are doing the opposite, your sleep will suffer—with immediate effect. Some will be more harmful than others. By questioning all your choices and all the information that led you to make those choices, you can identify which ones are most affecting your sleep and address those choices first.

So let's take a look at the common myths that fool us into sleep-disruptive lifestyle, behavioral, and diet choices, and begin to separate fact from fiction. Please continue to be patient when I use references to addictions such as alcohol and nicotine—as I've mentioned, if you don't drink or smoke, you can still relate the examples to your own food or drug consumption.

It's my personal choice

This is a popular argument among smokers, drinkers, gamblers etc—they'll all say things like, "You only get one life," or "You can't live forever," and claim that it's their personal right to do whatever they want to themselves during that one life.

But ask them when they consciously chose to become a permanent smoker, drinker, or gambler and they can't tell you. The simple truth is we no more choose to become these things than we choose to speak our native tongue. It is just part of the culture we are raised in.

We do choose to take the drug or partake in the addictive behavior in the first place, and we do choose to persevere until we can take the drug without feeling sick. But even that choice is heavily influenced by social pressure. By the time you're hooked, it's no longer a matter of choice but of addiction.

If smokers chose to keep smoking, why would they find it so difficult to stop? Smokers don't keep smoking out of choice, but because they aren't able to exercise their choice. The same is true of all addictions. Easyway is estimated to have helped 50 million people to freedom simply by making something that appeared hard and almost impossible into something easy. The clue is in the name.

I enjoy it

So-called problem gamblers claim to enjoy the thrill of betting. But have you ever studied one in the act? You might have noticed the intensity of their emotions, the heightened concentration, the almost machine-like way in which they place their bets. They don't savor each bet they place. There is no evidence of genuine pleasure each time they pump another coin into a slot machine, or try another throw of the dice, spin of the wheel, or turn the card. Each bet is swallowed up in the continuous frenzy of the whole gambling experience.

It's very similar to someone eating a chocolate bar. There is a rush to peel back the wrapper and take that first bite. Then the next bite, then the next, each mouthful barely finished before the next one is taken. In a matter of seconds the bar is devoured. There is no time taken savoring each mouthful; it is merely a race to eat the thing as quickly as possible. If it were genuine enjoyment, they'd take their time and savor it. It takes perseverance to build a resistance to the nauseous effects of nicotine and alcohol, both of which are highly toxic in their pure form. Like chocolate bars, most cigarettes and alcoholic drinks are consumed without giving a moment's thought to how they taste or smell. That's not the reason for consuming them. The reason is none other than to get the drug.

Smokers will argue that certain cigarettes are definitely more enjoyable than others. The first one of the day, one on vacation, or after sex, for example. How can an identical cigarette out of the same pack taste different just because of the occasion? The clue lies in the question: it's the occasion, not the cigarette.

The first one of the day feels special because you have gone for longer than usual without a fix. And a cigarette on vacation or after sex feels special because you are in a special situation. It's not the cigarette that makes it special. You're just scratching the itch, like you always do; you just happen to be in a particularly happy place. At that time a non-smoker feels fabulous without having to have a cigarette.

I like the ritual

Marketers are very conscious of this aspect of human nature. We like rituals, so they package their products in a way that adds a sense of anticipation to the act of consumption.

For smokers, this might be unwrapping a new pack, rolling a cigarette between your fingers, or flicking open your prized lighter. For drinkers, it could be pulling out the cork, decanting the wine, choosing the right glass, mixing the cocktail, or pouring the beer. Think about the rituals that go with your lifestyle choices and ask yourself why you really do them.

There is a lot to be said for rituals; they can undoubtedly add pleasure to life, but to claim they are the reason for smoking, drinking etc is nonsense. If you only did it for the ritual, why not just go through the ritual and then stop short of lighting the cigarette or drinking the drink?

It wouldn't be the same, would it? It would be like dining out without the food.

It relaxes me

The myth that addictive drugs and behaviors help you relax is explained in Chapter 5. After getting your fix, as the chemicals withdraw from your system, you become edgy and uptight. It's like having an itch you can't scratch.

When you have your next fix, you scratch that itch and feel some relief. It's like taking off tight shoes at the end of the day. The relief wouldn't come if it weren't for the discomfort that precedes it.

Because of the Big Monster, whenever you feel stressed or anxious for any reason, you think about the one thing that gives you relief from this uncomfortable feeling. You get a fix, the withdrawal and mental craving is partially relieved, and the myth that the fix fixed you is reinforced.

Meanwhile, the real cause of your stress or anxiety does not go away. If anything, it get worse because you're not doing anything about it. You're also doing further harm to yourself with each fix.

Feeling stressed and edgy from time to time in life is perfectly normal. For an addict, it is a permanent state.

It helps me concentrate
This one works along the same lines as the "It relaxes me" myth. The enemy of concentration is distraction. If there is something you can do to remove the distraction, then you will feel distracted and irritable until you have removed it. If there is nothing you can do about it, you accept it and move on.

It's true that many addicts find it impossible to concentrate without their drug, but that's only because they have the permanent "itch" and it will distract them until they are able to scratch it again—i.e. take another shot of the drug. As long as the drug is an option, they will fixate on it. Lock a smoker away in a room with no access to their cigarettes and they are able to concentrate, because they know that smoking is not an option.

It gives me confidence

This is the classic drinker's excuse, but it is used by other drug addicts too. They confuse confidence with lack of inhibition.

In social situations, self-consciousness can hold you back and prevent you from being yourself and talking freely. You see people who seem to have no problem finding things to say, and you want to have their confidence so you can join in. You drink to overcome the inhibition.

But inhibition serves a purpose. It is our way of keeping a watchful eye on our own behavior and avoiding doing or saying anything we'll later regret. Sure, it can feel smothering sometimes, but knocking it out with alcohol is like a pilot knocking out the aircraft's instruments when flying in fog over mountains. The danger doesn't go away, only your awareness of it.

Alcohol and other drugs do not give you anything. They create the impression of giving confidence by taking away your inhibitions.

This is dangerous on many levels. Knock out your inhibitions and what's to stop you from becoming oafish and obnoxious? What's to stop you from turning violent? What's to stop you from putting yourself in danger?

There is a way to overcome debilitating inhibitions, and that is to practice by putting yourself in social situations and staying sober. You will quickly learn how to let your personality shine through—and you will quickly notice that those confident talkers you aspired to be like are nothing more interesting than drunken loudmouths with no awareness of when to shut up and let someone else have a say.

I've got it under control

Addicts will always kid themselves that this is the case, because the alternative is too unpleasant to contemplate. Whenever they try to stop, though, it quickly becomes apparent that they are not in control; addiction is controlling them.

Accepting that you cannot control an addiction is a big step toward escaping from it. As long as you continue to get your fix, you will remain in the trap and sink further and further down.

I've been doing it for so long, I can't stop now

It's the old saying, "You can't teach an old dog new tricks." And with that resignation to the inevitable, some addicts labor through life wasting their money, damaging their health, and becoming more and more miserable and helpless.

The length of time you spend with an addiction does not affect your ability to quit. In fact, it's often the longer-term, heavier addicts who find it easier to stop than the younger, casual addicts. That's because the long-term addicts have lost the Illusion of Pleasure. They've been doing it so long, they know that all those excuses they used to make are nonsense, and that they are in a trap. They wish they could quit. All they need is the key to get out.

If there is something wrong in your life, you have a choice: keep on suffering as you are, or make a change. If it's something as serious as sleep deprivation, the only logical choice is to make a change.

It's not the best time right now

This is the final excuse of the addict who knows they need to quit but doesn't know how. They put it off until some landmark occasion, like New Year's Eve or their birthday.

But why wait to improve your life? Choosing a special day does not make it easier to quit; it's just an excuse for putting it off. It's a sign that you don't fully understand the trap you are in and have not removed the fear of success. Whatever you decide you need to change, the best time to do it is right now.

WIN THE TUG-OF-WAR

The excuses we make to keep our sleep-disruptive lifestyle choices, behaviors, and diet are evidence of the confusion that keeps us trapped. There is no logic in these excuses, and it only takes a little examination to see how unconvincing they really are.

We persist with the excuses because we are afraid of the changes we know we need to make. By seeing things as they really are and unraveling the brainwashing, you can begin to remove this fear and win the tug-of-war.

TRUST YOUR SENSES

Reconnecting with reality is as simple as making a conscious choice. Try not to consume mindlessly, as we've grown up doing.

Pay attention to how things taste, how they smell, how they feel, and how they make you feel.

What you feel is your senses working, rather than brain-washing. The Big Monster is beginning to die.

Enjoy the feeling of sitting with your senses. Take time. Relax. Make it part of your routine, every time you eat, drink, exercise, work, and entertain. Ask yourself, "Am I enjoying this? How does it feel? How does it taste?" You will notice your senses start to come alive again. The pathways get stronger. Question everything you do, why you do it, and how it makes you feel when you're doing it. You feel a new sense of power, like finding a tool in your garage that you thought you didn't have. Use it! It's designed for happiness.

Chapter 13

HOW MUCH SLEEP DO YOU NEED?

•THE IDEAL AMOUNT OF SLEEP •NATURAL SIGNALS
•NATURAL SIGNALS DURING THE DAY •NIGHT OWLS AND
MORNING PEOPLE •HOW TO SLEEP—THE THREE Cs

THE IDEAL AMOUNT OF SLEEP

As you begin to change your lifestyle, it helps to have a clear idea of what you're aiming for. How much sleep should you be getting and how will you know when you're getting it?

Sleep is part of the body's daily cycle, which needs to adhere to a consistent timetable for best results. The amount of sleep we need varies according to age and the extent to which we exert ourselves during the day. An athlete, for example, needs about an hour extra per night for full recovery.

Newborn babies need between 14 and 17 hours of sleep per night, but by the time they reach school age that falls to between nine and 11 hours. For most of our adult life, we should be trying to get between seven and nine hours' sleep per night, and in old age we can get by with about an hour less.

The difference between seven and nine hours is sizable. If you need nine hours and only get seven, that's just over two-thirds of the sleep you need. It's important to find your own personal sleep requirement and not rely on recommended figures.

Neither should you take that wide range to mean that it's healthy to get seven hours one night, nine the next, eight the next and so on. But you don't need to worry about that right now. There's a surefire way of telling when you're getting the sleep you need.

It's another example of the ingenuity of the Incredible Machine. The scientific study of sleep is a hot topic, and teams of researchers are constantly working to understand exactly how the sleep process happens and the factors that decide how much sleep we need. But members of remote tribes, who have never seen a medical journal in their life, manage to get the precise amount of sleep they need, every night of their lives, without anyone telling them how many hours they should be aiming for. How? By responding to their body's signals.

They go to sleep when they feel tired and wake up when fully refreshed.

That is what you should be aiming for. Your body will tell you how much sleep you need, and if you pay attention to the signals, you will fall into a regular sleep routine that is ideally suited to you and your physical and mental needs.

By paying attention to your body's signals, you will know when you are getting the right amount of sleep and when you are not. Eight hours is a useful guide, but when you restore your sleep to the ideal, natural pattern that Mother Nature designed for you, you might find you need nine hours or you might find you feel your best on seven.

It's important to get it right because, just as sleep deprivation leads to debilitating short-term and long-term health impacts, oversleeping has been shown to have a strong link to the same outcomes. There is an obvious reason for this. If you regularly sleep for more than nine hours, it's a sign that the sleep you are getting is not sufficiently high quality.

Remember the different stages of sleep we go through and how the different restorative processes take place during these stages? If your sleep is broken and disturbed, those restorative processes won't happen—or not as fully as they need to—so you will still feel that you haven't really rested after nine hours.

The most important thing is not the timetable you set for sleeping but the attention you pay to your body's signals. Trust in the Incredible Machine and it will set the timetable for you.

NATURAL SIGNALS

So what are these signals that you need to watch out for? Let's take a closer look at the symptoms of sleep problems and how you should respond to them.

Difficulty getting to sleep:

You go to bed feeling tired, but as soon as you turn out the light your mind seems to come alive. You feel desperate for sleep, but for some reason it doesn't come.

This can be due to a number of things. You may have a lot on your mind—worried or nervous about something you've got coming up, perhaps, or something you haven't done.

It can also be caused by the conditions in the room. Too stuffy? Too hot? Is the bed comfortable? Do you have too many pillows? Too few pillows? Personally, I had no idea how much better I would sleep with one less pillow.

If you are uncomfortable physically or mentally, you will find it difficult to get to sleep. While you're lying there, rather than wrestling with your inability to get to sleep, pay attention to how you're feeling, both in your body and in your mind, and you will identify where the disturbance is coming from.

Your mind may have been overstimulated, perhaps by caffeine or alcohol, or by looking at electronic devices just before trying to sleep. Some medications can also interfere with sleep. Remember, the chemical effects of stimulants disrupt sleep in a number of ways: they cause stress, over-stimulate your mental alertness, and impede your sleep hormones.

If you're regularly struggling to get to sleep, it's a sign that something is causing you physical or mental discomfort. Using the knowledge you have gained, figure out what it is and do something to change it.

Mid-sleep wakefulness:
Assuming you don't have an obvious physical pain that is keeping you awake, waking up in the middle of the night and not being able to get back to sleep is a sign of mental stress. The natural processes that get you to sleep have done their job, but something has woken you up and now you can't get back to sleep. It's infuriating—and the more frustrated you get, the less sleepy you feel.

Your mind is telling you to take action, but because it's the middle of the night, getting up and taking action feels like the last thing you should be doing. But lying awake worrying or getting annoyed that you can't sleep is only going to make matters worse.

You need to pay attention to what action your mind is telling you to take and then make a decision. If you're lying awake fretting about something you need to do at work the next day, for example, then you need to let go. There is nothing you can do about it now, so tell yourself you will address it in the morning when you're awake or, better still, when you're at work.

If that doesn't help your mind relax, and you're fretting about the fact that you can't get to sleep, then you need to take action. Get out of bed and go somewhere else, such as a comfortable chair in another room. Make a note of the issue you need to address at work—so you don't have to worry about whether you'll remember it, then read a book or magazine, listen to some calming music or just try meditating on a comforting thought for a little while.

If you are worried about becoming overwhelmed by all the things you have to do, making a list can really help. In fact, the best time to do this is before you go to bed, so that when you wake up you can tell yourself you've got it all under control and the worry won't keep you awake.

Often it's the fear that you've forgotten or overlooked something that keeps your mind on high alert. By doing a little planning before you go to sleep, you're much less likely to suffer from this worry.

Avoid doing anything that overstimulates your mind in the middle of the night, such as drinking caffeine, playing a game or trying to solve the problems of the day. Allow your mind to unwind, feel the stress subsiding and when you feel your eyelids drooping again, go back to bed.

It's important that you don't lie awake in bed for a long time for two reasons: first, you just become more stressed, so sleep becomes harder; and second, you build an association between bed and the inability to sleep. You need to see your bed as a place where you enjoy delightful, easy sleep, not nights of restlessness and worry.

Waking up often:
Many things can wake you from your sleep in the middle of the night: a noise, a light, physical discomfort, anxiety. As you go through the cycles of light sleep, you are more prone to being woken by a slight disturbance, such as a car going by or your cat coming through the cat flap. But these disturbances are fleeting and, if all other conditions are OK, you will fall back to sleep very quickly and maybe not even register being woken at all.

But other conditions can turn these slight disturbances into big disturbances. The need to urinate will wake you up, and that increases with alcohol and caffeine consumption. Alcohol also brings about longer periods of light sleep, thus increasing the likelihood of being woken by a disturbance.

Gas or indigestion can wake you up, and this becomes increasingly likely if you eat close to bedtime. Time your mealtimes to give yourself a few hours to digest before lying down to sleep at night, and resist the temptation to snack, particularly on foods that cause big fluctuations in your blood-sugar levels, such as refined sugar and processed/starchy carbs.

Anxiety will not only keep you awake at night, but also wake you up. You are more likely to have nightmares if you're anxious during the day, and you can also experience panic attacks that are severe enough to wake you up.

If you wake up frequently during the night, it could be a combination of any of these factors, or it could be one factor that is repeatedly disturbing your sleep. By paying attention to your natural signals, you will be able to identify the causes and do something about them.

Waking up too early:
Waking up before you've had a full night's sleep can be due to any of the factors above, but it might also be the timing of your sleep routine. If you plan to sleep until 7am but the sun rises at 6am, there may be light flooding into your bedroom, or the sound of birds and people starting their day.

It can also be a case of conditioning. Your mind may have become accustomed to waking up an hour earlier than you want to. If your body clock is waking you up at 6am rather than 7am, and telling you to get up and start your day, maybe you need to listen to it. If that doesn't give you the sleep you think you need, try going to bed an hour earlier.

Your body is trying to tell you something, and you won't solve your problem by ignoring it.

NATURAL SIGNALS DURING THE DAY

That is the golden rule: don't ignore the natural signals your body is sending you. The same rule applies during the day.

When you are awake, trying to think straight or work energetically, if your body and mind have not had sufficient sleep, they will let you know by making you behave in certain ways. We all recognize these behaviors as classic signs of tiredness, but we are better at recognizing them in others than in ourselves.

It's time to start seeing these symptoms in yourself.

Feeling negative and moody:

Tiredness makes you feel less positive and optimistic, and problems appear magnified. Are you making a lot of negative comments? Are you coming up with lots of reasons why not and no reasons why?

It makes sense. If you're lacking energy, your mind will find excuses to do nothing rather than look for reasons to act. On the other hand, a fully refreshed mind and body will relish the opportunity for action.

If you're struggling to conjure up enthusiasm, it's a sign that you're not getting enough sleep.

Feeling irritable:

Lack of sleep affects tolerance and the ability to empathize and see things from other people's point of view.

We even tend to blame our irritability on others. Rather than seeing it as a failing of our own, we become rude and impatient and get into a spiral of frustration by expecting everybody else to change when it's us who needs to change.

This is stressful and tiring, so the problem gets worse and worse. There are two ways it can end: in an argument, or by recognizing that you are irritable because you are tired, and doing something about getting more sleep. Apologizing for sleep-deprived moodiness can also help people cut you a little slack.

Having difficulty concentrating:
The work your mind has to do during the day is entirely dependent on the rest and restoration it receives at night. The better you sleep, the better you are able to concentrate.

We don't tend to see it that way, though. We seem to think we can force ourselves to concentrate. Think about the student who stays up all night studying, then wonders why the test didn't go as well as they had expected. There's no point filling your mind with facts if you're then too tired to recall them or arrange them into coherent answers.

The best preparation for a test is a great study plan and a good night's sleep. If you are finding it hard to concentrate, that is a signal that you have not slept enough, and your brain is still tired.

Of course, struggling to concentrate in a test is bad, but it's not life-threatening. Struggling to concentrate at the wheel of a car or truck, or while operating machinery, can very easily be fatal.

Craving junk food:
Poor sleep increases the tendency to crave junk food—the things

we regard as a reward, such as cake, chocolate bars, potato chips and cookies. This is inappropriately known as "comfort eating." This symptom goes hand-in-hand with those above because we wrongly believe these foods provide a pick-me-up.

Deep down we know that they are nothing of the kind, but an indulgence that we know is not good for us. It's only the belief that they give us some so-called "guilty pleasure" that makes us crave them. My book *Good Sugar Bad Sugar* explores the manipulation of blood-sugar levels, refined sugars' mimicking of natural foods that are good for us (fruit, for example), and the food industry's barefaced exploitative treatment of consumers by selling cheap, unnutritious, bland, unpleasant food (often processed and starchy carbs) by pumping it full of refined sugar, salt, and additives with addictive qualities.

How can something that causes you physical harm give you pleasure? It's the confusion of the brainwashed mind, and it's a common sign of sleep deficiency.

Constant anxiety:
Anxiety is a natural warning system designed to help us avoid potential dangers. Constant anxiety, however, is an unnatural state of permanent fear brought on by unclear thinking.

Anxiety increases with fatigue. If you find that you are feeling anxious a lot and you cannot rationalize your fears, it's a strong sign that your mind is not getting the sleep it needs to process your thoughts and restore itself. Anxiety and eating junk are easy signals to identify. Feeling moody or irritable, or having trouble concentrating are quite subtle signals that can be hard to detect in ourselves, especially if they become a long-term condition. So watch out for the more obvious outcomes that can result from these changes.

Relationships will start to break down. Your social life will suffer and friends will fall away. You won't look forward to work and you'll find it harder than usual. You'll find yourself eating more, particularly between meals, and avoiding exercise.

These are all signals that you are not getting enough sleep. You don't need a book to tell you how many hours to get. Your mind and body will tell you right away.

NIGHT OWLS AND MORNING PEOPLE— THE CIRCADIAN RHYTHM

We explained in Chapter 2 how light and dark affect the sleep function. Your body has a waking mechanism that is controlled by daylight and a sleeping mechanism that is controlled by darkness.

But unless you live on the Equator, it is impractical in the modern world to live by the sun. It would mean keeping very different hours in winter and summer. Of course, that's what wild animals do, but we are not wild animals, and we have arranged our way of life to keep regular hours year-round.

To help us do this we have a body clock, which regulates many functions, such as sleep, digestion, cell building, body temperature etc. The body clock likes to keep regular time. It is known as the Circadian rhythm, and not everybody's is the same. That's why you get "morning people" and "night owls."

Some people are just more suited to early starts; others operate better at night.

The important thing is to live in time with your body clock. Are you a morning person? Then you might need to go to bed a little earlier in order to get the full night's sleep you need. If you're a night owl, you'll need to compensate for those late nights by waking up later.

The problem arises when a night owl has to get up early for work, or a morning person has to work late. It's a very common occurrence and it helps explain why there is an insomnia epidemic. Millions of people are fighting their body clocks. Having said that, we are hugely adaptable, and we can flex between early and late nights without too many issues.

Therefore, we cannot put all the blame on our work schedules. We make lifestyle choices that fight our body clocks. We eat late, stay up late, and stimulate ourselves with caffeine and digital devices late into the evening.

Some people have to work irregular shifts, and that is a major obstacle to sleep, but if they follow a good sleep plan, it can be overcome. Most of us, however, have a regular daytime schedule, which allows plenty of time between finishing work and starting again the next day in which to eat, digest, relax, and get a good night's sleep, with enough margin to align with our body clocks much better than we currently do.

Take the standard 9 to 5. Say you have a one-hour commute to work and a one-hour commute home: that means leaving the house at 8am and returning at 6pm. That leaves time to cook and eat your evening meal by 7.30pm, relax and unwind for three hours, get ready for bed, go to sleep at 11pm, and wake up at 7am, fully refreshed, with an hour to get ready to go.

You might protest, "But I work longer hours than that!" "My commute takes an hour and a half!" "I don't want to go to sleep at 11pm!"This is where you need to examine your lifestyle choices. If your work means you have to leave the house at 5am and don't get home until 7pm, that still leaves 10 hours at home. Take out eight hours' sleep and you're left with one hour on either side.

Now that might not be your idea of an exciting lifestyle, but it should be the absolute basis for everything else you choose to do. Unless you put sleep at the top of your list of priorities EVERY DAY, you will continue to suffer from sleep problems.

When you know the long-term effects of chronic sleep deprivation, a good night's sleep should be non-negotiable. It's everything around it that needs to adapt. That could mean negotiating different work hours; preparing meals in advance so you spend less time cooking and more time relaxing; moving to a job that is closer to home, or working from home.

When you stop and think about it, losing sleep because you spend three hours a day traveling to and from work is illogical.

Rearrange your daily schedule to give yourself the sleep you need. Then you can see what you feel you are missing out on and make adjustments accordingly. For example, if you like to play tennis one evening a week, go for it, but allow your usual schedule to snap back to normal on other nights. Always pay attention to the signals. Adjust your sleep schedule to align with your body clock and give you the precise amount of sleep you need. Your body will tell you when you've got it right.

HOW TO SLEEP—THE THREE Cs

Sleep hygiene is the popular term used for creating the ideal environment for healthy sleep. It includes your routine, your activities, and the physical environment in which you sleep. To help you remember the key elements of sleep hygiene, use the three Cs:

Consciousness

Consistency

Comfort

Follow these tips to create the ideal sleep environment.

Consciousness:

Place sleep at the top of your priorities.

Be aware of the sleep-disruptive effects of stimulants, drugs, and electronic devices and the enhancing benefits of exercise and good diet. Adjust your lifestyle accordingly.

Quit smoking.

Limit alcohol consumption to weekends.

Keep your phone and other devices out of the bedroom.

Avoid caffeine after 11am.

Do regular exercise at a time that suits you.

Avoid eating before going to bed.

Be prepared for nighttime anxieties by thinking about the next day's tasks and concerns before bedtime and having a strategy planned.

Consistency:

Create a consistent sleep routine that begins first thing in the morning. Plan your daily timetable to enable you to wind down and go to bed at the same time every night, including weekends, allowing for the amount of sleep you need.

Start by allowing for eight hours and adjust gradually until you feel aligned with your body clock.

Sleep in the same bed every night. Unfamiliar surroundings put your brain on alert.

Try to eat your evening meal at least three hours before bedtime.

Build in an hour without devices before bedtime.

Give yourself a relaxing pre-bed routine, e.g. bath, read, listen to the radio, meditate.

Comfort:

Remove anything that causes physical discomfort during sleep. Make your bed a haven. Choose a good mattress and comfortable pillows and bedding. Go to the bathroom before bed.

Make sure the room is dark during the hours you plan to sleep and do what you can to minimize noise disturbances.

Bathe before bed. Your body temperature needs to fall by 1.8°F to induce sleep, so raising it first in the shower or bath helps this process.

Set the room temperature no higher than 64°F.

More than anything, put sleep at the top of your list of priorities. After water and food, sleep is the most important thing your body needs. Let your body set the timetable and then follow it every day.

Chapter 14

BE KIND TO YOURSELF

The three Cs — Consciousness, Consistency, and Comfort — give you a framework for planning your daily routine around a good night's sleep. While most sleep therapy advice you will come across focuses on the second and third of these, it's actually the first, Consciousness, that is the most important of all.

Consciousness concerns the lifestyle choices that create the right conditions for a good night's sleep. Until now, we have looked at this from the opposite angle: the lifestyle choices we make that disrupt our sleep. We did this to highlight the number of traps you can fall into unwittingly.

It's important to be aware of the traps so you can avoid them, or break free of them if you are already trapped.

But now let's look at these lifestyle choices from the positive side. The fourth instruction was to begin with a feeling of elation. That feeling is fueled by the thought of all the benefits you will enjoy, not only from curing your sleep problem but also from the positive lifestyle choices you will make in achieving that.

The first is all about diet: the food, drugs, and drinks you choose to consume.

A SLEEP-HEALTHY DIET

Do you ever ask yourself why you eat? It might seem like a strange question. Obviously, if you didn't eat you would starve to death. But that is not what you're thinking every time you eat, is it? "I have to eat dinner or I will starve to death." In fact, the most common drivers for eating are:

Routine
Temptation
Boredom
Restlessness
Sociability

There is nothing wrong with eating according to a routine. It's practical and it generally fits in with your body clock. But if the routine is too rigid it can cause a problem.

The actual reason you eat is to give the body the fuel it needs to fulfill the multitude of functions it performs. In this respect it is very much like a car. Do you fuel your car by putting in the same amount at the same time every day? If you did there would be times when the fuel tank overflowed, spilling gas all over the place!

To help us know when the car needs fuel, manufacturers provide us with a fuel gauge. Wouldn't it be easy if Mother Nature did the same? Well, guess what—she does! Your body has a fuel gauge: it's called hunger.

Hunger is the signal that your body is running low on nutrients and needs to refuel. For a sleep-healthy diet, you need to pay attention to your natural fuel gauge, just as you would pay attention to the gauge in your car.

When you eat the same quantity every day at the same time because that is your routine, or you eat because you're craving sugar and a piece of cake looks tempting, or you eat because you're bored or restless, or because it's a social occasion and there's lots of food and everyone else is going for it—when you eat for these reasons, chances are you are overfilling the tank.

The excess spills over as fat. Then we try to lose it by exercising or going on a diet and depriving ourselves for a while. Weight becomes a source of physical discomfort, stress, and anxiety, leading to sleep loss.

Remember, the hunger gauge indicates the level of vital nutrients in your body, not the quantity of food you've put in your stomach. When the level is low, you feel hungry. Eat foods that are low in nutrients and you will keep feeling hungry. In order to get the nutrients you need and top up the gauge, you have to eat more, create more waste and build up more fat.

This drains your energy, making you feel tired even when you haven't exerted yourself. And it makes it harder to sleep at night.

When you eat in response to hunger, you stop when the tank is full. Chances are you will still eat according to a regular routine because that is how your body clock works, but the types of food you eat and the quantity will vary according to the amount you're burning off.

When you eat nutritious foods—particularly fruit, vegetables and nuts—the hunger gauge quickly registers full with very little waste. The food tastes great, leaves you feeling revitalized and brimming with energy, and it doesn't overflow as fat. You don't have to bother with diets or vigorous exercise to burn off fat; all you have to think about is your intake of fuel.

So the recipe for a sleep-healthy diet is to eat nutritious foods when hungry and stop when not. Eat slowly, savor the flavor, and notice the gauge responding.

The reason for eating slowly is to allow for the lag while your body absorbs the nutrients it needs and this registers on the fuel gauge. With fruit, vegetables, and nuts, this happens much more quickly than with meat and other heavy foods, which take a long time to digest.

THE JUNK MARGIN

In case you're thinking you have to become a vegan and give up all your favorite foods in order to cure your sleep problem, rest assured that is not the case. We've recommended fruit, vegetables, seeds, and nuts because those are the foods that Mother Nature designed for us to eat. They are the most nutritious, the easiest to digest, and they also happen to be the tastiest.

Remember, taste is the sense we are given to help us identify the foods that are best for us to eat. We have largely lost touch with this connection because the food industry has brainwashed us into believing that processed foods with high sugar and salt content are those we like best. The good news is that this natural connection between taste and nutritional benefit can be quickly rebuilt when you pay attention to your senses while eating.

But you don't have to stick solely to fruit, vegetables, seeds, and nuts. Mother Nature allowed us some margin, so that our ancestors could live off of other foods when their favorite foods were not available. Thanks to this, they evolved with the ability to eat meat and some roots, which needed to be cooked to make them edible, but gave our ancestors sufficient nutrients to survive when more nutritious foods were scarce.

Thanks to this margin, we can eat all kinds of foods today and still survive. Our bodies have the ability to digest a wide variety of foods—it's just that some take more time and energy than others, and we have to eat more of them to get the nutrients we need.

Thanks to this ability of the Incredible Machine, you don't have to sacrifice anything from your diet. You can keep eating all your favorite foods. All you need to adjust is the proportion.

I call this the Junk Margin. As long as your diet is mostly nutritious foods, you can allow yourself anything you like in your Junk Margin. The problem is that the brainwashing has tipped the balance the wrong way, so we eat mostly junk and very little nutritious food. Foods that were supposed to be secondary options when our favorite foods were scarce are now the basis of the modern diet.

For a sleep-healthy diet, you need to pay attention to the balance of your diet and make sure you are eating mostly nutritious foods. You will quickly start to feel the benefits in terms of energy, weight, and sleep. Furthermore, as you reconnect your senses with your eating, you will start to recognize that nutritious foods are actually the tastiest, and your craving for junk will diminish.

This is a natural process that happens gradually. Unlike dieting, which forces an abrupt change on your body and leaves you feeling deprived, focusing on nutritious foods while allowing yourself a Junk Margin means eating and drinking remains a pleasure—in fact, it becomes more of a pleasure over time.

EXERCISE FOR PLEASURE

When talking about excess weight and fat burning, I may have created the impression that you should not exercise. That was not the intention.

Exercise is a major benefit to sleep and to a healthy lifestyle in general. But exercise, like eating, should be a pleasure. To prove the point, the body actually produces chemicals that make us feel good after exercise.

Exercising to lose weight is a different matter. It's like driving your car just to burn off fuel. The motivation is flawed. Feeling overweight is a negative mindset, and the exercise we do to try to lose weight tends to feel more like a punishment—the "no pain, no gain" mentality.

How much of your life do you want to spend punishing yourself? When you eat a sleep-healthy diet, you don't need to punish yourself at all, because your diet takes care of your weight.

It is all in balance. It's when you overdo the junk that things get out of balance.

The eighth instruction is:

Exercise only for pleasure.

There are two important reasons for this. The first is that the pursuit of pleasure is what we are trying to achieve with your sleep cure. The second is that choosing a form of exercise that you enjoy will mean you stick with it, and it becomes part of your lifestyle.

This doesn't happen when you exercise to lose weight. You push yourself to burn off the pounds and then, once you get down to your target weight, you reward yourself by giving up the exercise and going back to your previous lifestyle. Surprise surprise, the weight piles back on.

"Exercise only for pleasure" is not a difficult instruction to follow. There are innumerable choices when it comes to exercise, and they are all designed to be fun, as long as you're not doing them just to lose weight.

Research has shown that exercise helps with both getting to sleep and getting the quality of sleep you need. It is particularly beneficial for deep sleep. We know that exercise raises your body temperature, and when it falls again that induces sleepiness. It's the same effect as having a bath before bedtime.

Some people, however, find that doing exercise in the late evening keeps them awake. This could be because of the chemicals the body produces during exercise, called endorphins, which stimulate the brain and make you feel wide awake and happy.

Another hormone released during exercise is serotonin, which regulates your mood and controls the sleep-wake cycle. The production of these hormones through exercise helps alleviate stress and anxiety, putting you in a more relaxed mental state, which naturally aids sleep.

And, of course, while weight loss should not be your motivation, the effect of exercise on weight is a further benefit to sleep. People who do regular exercise as part of their lifestyle are less prone to obesity, which is a major cause of sleep disorders.

HOW AND WHEN TO EXERCISE

The amount of exercise you do and the time of day when you choose to do it are entirely up to you. There is no one-size-fits-all.

The more you enjoy exercise, the more you will want to do it. The more you do, the more fuel you will burn off. The more fuel you burn off, the hungrier you will feel. The hungrier you feel, the more nutritious food you will eat. The more nutrients you consume, the more exercise you will be capable of doing.

It's a wonderful cycle, and it works in any quantity. Do a little exercise and you won't feel so hungry. You will eat smaller portions, still get the nutrients you need, and maintain a healthy body.

Your body will tell you when and how much to exercise. Some people are capable of running marathons, others are better suited to a walk or some light exercises indoors. Some people find exercising first thing in the morning sets them up for the day and improves their sleep, but others find that evening exercise is more beneficial.

Again, you have the tools to make your own decisions. Listen to your body and pay attention to your sleep patterns. Through trial and error you will learn how much exercise you enjoy and what time of day gives you the most benefit at night. If you're worried that you have to become an athlete—forget it!—a brisk 30-minute walk three times a day is all you really need.

KEEP IT REGULAR

How often do you wake up before your alarm goes off? Even when you change your alarm to 4am because you have to catch a flight, say, it's common to wake up before it goes off. Your mind just seems to know, doesn't it?

The body clock is an incredibly sophisticated function, and the above is an example of how it manages our physical and mental processes without us being conscious of the fact.

You can think of the body clock as a multitude of different clocks, each regulating different parts of the body. It works best when all those clocks are in sync.

So while your mental clock might wake you up at 4am to catch your flight, the rest of your body is not in sync, and you feel very tired as you drag yourself out of bed. That tiredness will catch up with you later in the day, or even a day or two later, as the body clock readjusts.

For healthy sleep, it is important to keep the body clock as consistent and regular as you can. That means getting into routines. When you go to bed, when you get up, when you work, when you unwind, when you exercise.

We mentioned earlier that when you eat should be dictated by hunger, not routine. That is absolutely true. But as you build a routine for all the other activities in your life, hunger will align with your body clock and you will find that you feel the need to eat at the same times every day.

You will notice that we said "when you go to bed" and "when you get up," not "when you sleep" and "when you wake." That's because the sleep-wake cycle is controlled by the body clock. All you can do is create the ideal conditions for sleep and make sure you're in a position to sleep when the clock is ready.

By keeping to a regular routine, you will find this easy. Be prepared to make adjustments as you pay attention to your body's signals. Perhaps you're lying in bed for a while before falling asleep and could comfortably go to bed later. Nothing should be set in stone from the outset, but as you find the routine that works for you, make it consistent.

With your body clock in sync, you won't even have to think about it any more. Sleep will come naturally, night after night.

No need to wait

You don't have to wait until you reach this blissful state before you can tell yourself that you've beaten your sleep problem. As you make the changes you need to create the ideal conditions for sleep, you will see the improvements right away. There is nothing to wait for.

It's important that you don't feel impatient to reach the stage when you don't have to think about it any more. It's absolutely fine to be conscious of your sleep problem—you need to pay attention to the signals your body is sending you.

The difference is that now, when you think about sleep, rather than feeling anxious and telling yourself, "Oh no, I'm going to have another broken night," you can feel elated and remind yourself, "I'm no longer an insomniac; I am in control of my sleep, and it will just keep getting better every day!"

Chapter 15

REVERSING ADDICTIONS

•QUESTION THE ILLUSION OF PLEASURE
•EXERCISE YOUR SENSES •YOU ARE NOT GIVING
UP ANYTHING •SUBSTITUTES •KILLING THE MONSTERS

QUESTION THE ILLUSION OF PLEASURE

According to the willpower method, quitting smoking and other sleep-disruptive issues means fighting with all your will to resist the temptation to continue with something you regard as a pleasure or crutch. With Easyway, there is no need to fight, because you remove that temptation altogether.

The temptation is based on an illusion—the Illusion of Pleasure. People find it hard to quit addictive drugs and behaviors because they believe it means sacrificing something that they truly enjoy and depend on, and they believe that the process of quitting is hard and miserable. Both beliefs are myths.

Nobody smokes for pleasure. They do it because nicotine is highly addictive, and it keeps them coming back for more. There may be aspects of the ritual of smoking that they think they enjoy, but then why not follow the ritual without actually smoking the cigarette? Without the fix, there is no Illusion of Pleasure.

This is true of all addictions. We make excuses for why we continue with behaviors that we know are harmful to us and disrupt our sleep, but these excuses are just a cover for the real reason—it's addiction that keeps us coming back for more.

Addiction creates the Illusion of Pleasure by first making you uncomfortable (the Little Monster), then partially relieving the discomfort. At the same time, it brainwashes you into believing that it is the only thing that can relieve the discomfort (the Big Monster).

Without taking the drug in the first place, you would not experience the restless, uneasy sensation of withdrawal. If you don't wear tight shoes, you won't suffer from sore feet. Sure, you won't experience the relief of taking them off, but would you deliberately wear tight shoes for this reason?

When you take a conscious approach to your lifestyle choices, you begin to see through the Illusion of Pleasure. When you understand how addiction works, you begin to realize that the only thing really making you believe you don't want to change your lifestyle choices is the trap. This is how you kill the Big Monster—by seeing through the illusions and understanding that these lifestyle choices do nothing for you at all. You only do them because they are addictive.

Once you see through the Illusion of Pleasure and kill the Big Monster, it's easy to kill the Little Monster. You just have to starve it of its fix. As soon as you quit, you break the cycle of addiction because you are no longer feeding the two monsters. You escape the trap. It really is that straightforward.

By stopping to question everything you consume and every way in which you spend your time, you give your natural survival mechanism the chance to guide you. This is the conscious approach. You reconnect with your senses, and by paying heed to what your Incredible Machine is telling you, rather than your intellect and that of everybody who has ever influenced you, you unravel the brainwashing and start seeing things as they really are.

At the same time, you begin to feel the benefits of your new lifestyle choices. You feel fitter and healthier from eating nutritious foods; you feel pleasure and alertness from exercising; and you feel all the wonderful, restorative benefits of a good night's sleep.

Most importantly, you regain control. Addiction gives you the illusion of control, but deep down you know you are being controlled. This creates confusion and self-loathing—two stressful mental states that are hugely disruptive of sleep. You will know when you are truly in control of your lifestyle choices—there will be clarity in your decisions and your self-esteem will rise. Now your mind is in an ideal state for untroubled sleep.

EXERCISE YOUR SENSES

You may be wondering what exactly we mean by reconnecting with your senses and how you should go about it. Perhaps you feel you are already connected—you can smell things, you can taste things… all your senses seem to be working just fine.

That's great, but are you really paying attention to what they are telling you? We are so conditioned to believe what we are told, rather than what we sense for ourselves, that the connection with our senses has become weak. You can strengthen the connection the same way you strengthen any other facet of the Incredible Machine—through practice.

Walking is a great way to exercise both your body and your senses. As you walk, pay attention to the world around you. Notice the sounds, the smells, the colors, and the shapes. Feel the ground under your feet and the air on your hands and face.

You can exercise your senses on any walk. It doesn't have to be somewhere serene or picturesque, like the countryside or the beach. A walk to the store, or from the bus stop to the office, offers the same opportunities for connecting with your senses.

Most of us walk around without really paying attention to what's going on around us. Often we walk with our eyes on the ground, lost in thought. Walking is very good for thinking, too, by the way. It helps you de-stress by giving you time and space to reflect and come up with plans and solutions.

But remember, your brain is a computer—a very powerful one—and it works by analyzing data, which it gathers from various sensors: your eyes, your ears, your nose, your taste buds, your skin. The more data it can gather, the more informed its thinking and the better the solutions it will come up with.

So when you're walking, keep your head up and pay attention to everything you see; you will notice that your brain feels more alert and quick to make connections between all the information it's taking in. You will also remember more.

Do you ever have that feeling when you're driving somewhere that you can't remember anything about the last five minutes at the wheel? You wonder how you managed to keep going without getting into an accident, because it feels like your mind has been completely switched off. The human mind has the power to do this when performing familiar tasks; it can shut off conscious thought but still respond as normal, or even better, to the information coming in through the senses, like a kind of autopilot.

The only downside is that your experiences pass you by without getting logged in your memory. If someone asked you the name of the school you just drove past, you probably wouldn't even remember that you drove past a school.

We spend a lot of our waking time in this state of mind, automatically performing familiar tasks. And we pursue sleep-disruptive lifestyle choices in the same state of mind, responding only to the demands of the Little Monster, rather than paying attention to how they are really making us feel.

It's very easy to change this. You just need to make a conscious decision to do so. Practice when you are walking, eating, socializing and doing any other activity you enjoy. Bring your senses to the party. Use them to get the most from the experience. And listen to the signals when they sound a warning.

YOU ARE NOT GIVING UP ANYTHING

We have made the point throughout this book that you don't need willpower to bring about the lifestyle changes necessary to cure your sleep problem. In fact, relying on willpower is doomed to failure.

You only need to apply willpower when you have a conflict of wills. When you decide to change your lifestyle for the better, why would any part of your brain send a message to prevent you from doing that? That would only happen if you believed you were making a sacrifice—giving up some sort of pleasure or crutch. If that were the case, you would need constant willpower every day in order to resist the temptation to relapse.

That is why the willpower method is always doomed to failure. It only deals with the Little Monster. It does not remove the illusion that you are making a sacrifice, so you are constantly battling the desire to continue. At the same time, you are feeling deprived and sorry for yourself because you can't have your little crutch. Even if your willpower holds out for the rest of your life, you will always suffer from this feeling of deprivation.

Most people do not hold out. Their willpower eventually cracks, and they are dragged back into the trap, more firmly imprisoned than before because they have just proven to themselves that escape is impossible.

It's essential that you do not feel you are making sacrifices in any new lifestyle choices that you are making to cure your sleep problem. There can be no conflict of wills. The conscious approach helps remove any illusion that you are "giving up" anything.

Get it clear in your mind that the changes you are making are purely for the better. Anything that disrupts your sleep is your enemy, and the only reason you might think otherwise is because you have been brainwashed. But you have come a long way toward unraveling the brainwashing. You should now understand how addiction cons you into thinking you need things that actually do you nothing but harm, and how keeping sight of this fact will allow you to see through the illusions that keep you trapped.

When talking about your lifestyle changes, avoid the phrase

"giving up," even if you are just talking to yourself. "Giving up" implies a sacrifice, but this is not a sacrifice; it's shaking off the bonds that have kept you trapped and unable to sleep properly. That is a great feeling. It is freedom.

SUBSTITUTES

There is a flawed theory that suggests using substitutes to help conquer addictions. It's very important that you don't fall for this approach.

The theory is widely promoted by so-called experts, and it sounds pretty logical, in principle: in order to stop smoking, say, you replace cigarettes with a cleaner form of the drug, such as nicotine patches or e-cigarettes, so you stop inhaling the fumes right away while you concentrate on weaning yourself off the drug. Then you reduce the dose of the substitute bit by bit until you find it easy to quit completely. The harm-reduction aspects of vaping as opposed to smoking are positive; however, it is becoming increasingly clear that the idea behind it involves continued nicotine addiction for the rest of the addict's life, incurring a lifetime of cost, health worries, control, and slavery.

But can you spot the flaw in that, and in substitutes in general? In fact, there are two reasons why substitutes don't hold up.

1. The physical effects of withdrawal are negligible—nothing worse than a slight itch. So there is no reason to keep using the drug.

2. As long as you keep using the drug you will need all your willpower to reduce the dose, because the effect of addiction is to always want more.

Using a substitute might silence the Little Monster for a while, but it does nothing to kill the Big Monster. In fact, it helps keep the Big Monster alive. Twenty years ago, e-cigarettes didn't exist. Now millions of people are hooked on them. Clearly they are not helping people quit nicotine. In fact, they are adding to nicotine addiction by making it easier to get your fix (you can use e-cigarettes in places where smoking is prohibited) and lulling people into the belief that it is safe.

It may be less harmful than smoking; it is certainly not harmless. Nicotine is a highly toxic, highly addictive drug, and it has a serious impact on sleep.

We use the example of nicotine to show how substitutes are not helpful in overcoming addictions. Like the willpower method with which they are widely prescribed, they perpetuate the belief that you are trying to "give up" something. Whether you are substituting one form of the same drug with another, as in the case of e-cigarettes, or substituting one addiction for another, e.g. eating candy whenever you want a drink or cigarette, they keep the Big Monster alive.

KILLING THE MONSTERS

Without the Big Monster conning you into thinking you need your little crutch, killing the Little Monster is easy. All you need to do is starve it of its fix and in a few days it will be gone. We will look at this in more detail in Chapter 17 and explain why so many people believe that withdrawal is hard and painful, and something to be feared.

You're well on your way to killing the Big Monster. When you understand the truth, you don't need substitutes or willpower to overcome addictions and change your lifestyle choices for the better. You don't even have to <u>do</u> anything. All it takes is to <u>not</u> do something—keep feeding the Little Monster—and very soon any cravings will disappear.

Meanwhile, you can get on with your life, happy in the knowledge that you are regaining control and making great progress toward restoring your sleep pattern to where it needs to be.

Chapter 16

TAKING CONTROL

If you have skipped straight to this part of the book without reading anything that has gone before, sorry, but this chapter will not help you.

Up to this point we have been preparing the ground for creating the ideal conditions for sleep. Without reading the whole book, you will not have prepared the ground, and the plan we are going to look at in this chapter alone will not provide the cure. Please go back to the start and read the whole book. That is all you are required to do. The rest is easy.

If you have read everything up to this point, good! You will know that you are fully prepared. Don't worry if you don't feel ready—all you need to do is keep reading and follow the instructions, and you cannot fail.

Good sleep is essential for health and happiness. In fact, it is one of the most important requirements of all. When you find it difficult to get to sleep, or you wake in the night and struggle to get back to sleep, the cause is almost certainly something in the way you live your life.

This is great news, because it means you don't have to keep suffering from a lack of sleep and worrying about the long-term effects it could cause. You can do something about it.

By now you should be pretty clear about this. Your sleep problem is not something you are lumbered with. It has nothing to do with your genetic makeup or your personality. And while you may feel controlled by insomnia, this is not a permanent state that you will have to put up with for the rest of your life. You are in a position to retake control.

Hopefully you have identified the lifestyle choices, behavior, and dietary choices that have been preventing you from creating the ideal conditions for healthy sleep, and you have started to do something about changing them.

This requires a completely open mind. If you have followed all the instructions, you have kept an open mind about everything you have read so far, and you will understand that things you used to regard as a pleasure or a crutch are actually addictions that enslave you and keep you in an ingenious trap.

You will now understand the nature of addiction and how the trap works. It explains why we are so reluctant to "give up" things we know are harmful. By now you should have no doubt that you are not being asked to "give up" anything. On the contrary, you are making wonderful gains by changing these lifestyle choices. You are freeing yourself from the harmful physical effects that could trigger a critical health problem at any time. You are freeing yourself from the fear of that outcome. You are freeing yourself from the feeling of slavery and confusion that comes with being trapped. And by freeing yourself from these physical and mental impacts, you are giving yourself the freedom of good sleep.

THREE STEPS TO FREEDOM

Ingenious though it is, the trap has one fatal flaw: as the prisoner, you hold the key to your own release. In order to escape, you just need three things to happen:

1. You must recognize that you're in a trap

2. You must recognize that you hold the key

3. You must be shown how to use the key

This is how Easyway works. Everything you have read so far was designed to help you see the trap you're in and recognize that you hold the key.

The trap is a subtle combination of brainwashing causing the adoption of poor behavioral, lifestyle, and diet choices, many of which involve addiction. Whether you like the word or not, it is addictive substances that pose the biggest threat to sleep. Change your intake of these substances and you will take a big step toward creating the ideal conditions for sleep. You should by now feel fully prepared to do that.

The key is unraveling the brainwashing that keeps you addicted—killing the Big Monster. You do this by questioning if everything you have been told is true and identifying the truth by reconnecting with your senses and the signals your body sends you. Once you see through the illusions, you can never be fooled by them again.

The final step is to turn the key—to kill the Little Monster—and walk free. We will look at that in more detail in the next chapter.

These are the three steps to taking control of your lifestyle choices and getting rid of anything that disrupts your sleep. Killing the Little Monster simply means making different choices—choices that you make happily and of your own free will, not choices that are forced on you by peer pressure and the slavery of addiction.

THE MOMENT OF REVELATION

So how do you know when you're cured?

You win the tug-of-war the moment you kill the Big Monster. What does it feel like? It varies. Some describe it as a "eureka" moment—when everything clicks into place and the truth appears in sharp focus.

We call it the Moment of Revelation. You have given yourself the power to see what is really there, and it's a power that you can really enjoy.

Other people say they don't notice the Moment of Revelation, but they are completely clear about the truth and they can confidently say that they have killed the Big Monster. They feel in control.

If that is you, congratulations! You don't need fireworks and fanfares to tell you when you've killed the Big Monster. You just know. You see things differently. You notice things you didn't notice before. There is no confusion. If you remain unsure, please don't worry... you are getting there.

Whatever your experience of killing the Big Monster, you can celebrate your triumph and continue to finish the job, living your life the way you want to live it. You don't have to wait for the Little Monster to die. That will happen in a matter of days, and you will barely notice it.

You can stop thinking about it and focus instead on creating a sleep/wake routine that meets your requirements. Finalize your action list.

A NEW SLEEP ROUTINE

It's time to make a plan for how you are going to achieve the healthy night's sleep you need. It's helpful to write down a timetable so you can follow it every night, and when you make adjustments, you can keep a record of what worked best. Remember, you have diet, behavioral, and lifestyle decisions to make. Keep two separate documents: a list and a timetable.

ZERO HOUR

The optimum amount of sleep for an adult is between seven and nine hours. So let's split that down the middle and begin with eight. You know what time you need to wake up to be ready for work or whatever you have to do in the morning; count back eight hours and that is the time you need to go to sleep. We'll call this time zero hour. Remember, this is not bedtime, this is the time you need to be falling asleep.

ZERO MINUS 30

Thirty minutes before your scheduled sleep time, begin your wind-down. Take a hot bath or shower and go to bed with a book or something soothing on the radio. Alternatively, lie in bed and meditate. The important thing is that you are not doing anything stimulating or agitating.

Set the bedroom temperature no higher than 64°F. Go to the bathroom. Place a glass of water by the bed in case you wake up feeling thirsty. Make sure you are truly comfortable in bed. It should feel completely cozy and comforting. If anything is imperfect, fix it. Trying to get to sleep when you're not entirely comfortable is not the ideal start.

When you're ready, turn out the light. Practice steady breathing, in through the nose, out through the mouth, and allow your mind to relax and drift off to sleep.

ZERO MINUS 1 HOUR

An hour before your scheduled sleep time, switch off all digital devices and take them out of the bedroom. Look ahead to tomorrow and write down any tasks or concerns that are making you feel anxious. Plan how you are going to tackle those tasks and concerns the next day. If it means calling someone, put it on your list to make that call. If it means hunkering down and thinking through a problem, decide when will be the best time of day and the best place to do that.

The important thing is that you not start grappling with these challenges before bed, and that you go to bed knowing that you have a plan in place. This will give you peace of mind, in case you wake up worrying in the middle of the night.

ZERO MINUS 3 HOURS

Try to be done with your evening meal. Try to avoid eating after this time, and definitely don't drink alcohol.

If you prefer to exercise in the evening, you have the next two hours in which to do so.

ZERO MINUS 12 HOURS

Avoid any caffeine after this time.

ZERO MINUS 16 HOURS

Wake-up time. Once you are awake, try to get out of bed as soon as possible and start your day. Eat a healthy breakfast with plenty of fruit and nuts. If you prefer to exercise in the morning, build it into this time.

This is a basic schedule that prioritizes the time you need to spend asleep and works backward from there. You might want to add your own details, and you will probably make adjustments once you feel your body and mind responding to the new routine.

If you find yourself waking up refreshed after less than eight hours, try moving your zero hour later. If, on the other hand, you still don't feel refreshed after eight hours, move your zero hour earlier.

Make your adjustments gradually—say, five minutes at a time—and give yourself a few days after each adjustment to see how you respond over time. Those adjustments are the fine-tuning you need to get your sleep schedule in perfect sync with your body clock. It's necessary to be flexible and pay attention to how you are feeling, but remember the importance of consistency. Wild variations in your sleep routine are not what you need.

WHAT TO DO WHEN YOU WAKE

Even though you have prepared your mind and body for a good night's sleep, anything can disturb you during your sleep time. This is normal, and you need to be prepared for it.

If you do wake up in the middle of the night, instead of telling yourself, "Here we go again! Another night ruined," stay calm, remind yourself that waking in the night is perfectly normal and there is nothing to fret about. If anxious thoughts about the next day start whirring around your mind, tell yourself it's OK, you have a plan prepared, and you will deal with those anxieties in the morning.

If you find yourself trying to grapple with a problem while you lie awake, get up, and if you have another room, go there; if not, move to your chair/beanbag. You don't want bed to become associated with restless thoughts, and the longer you lie there awake, the more likely you are to get into a pattern of wakefulness.

Take yourself away, make sure you're warm, and occupy yourself with something relaxing, like reading a book. When you start to feel sleepy again, go back to bed.

If you were disturbed by a noise or light, make sure it doesn't happen again. If necessary, try wearing ear plugs and/or an eye mask to create the silence and darkness you need.

WHAT TO DO WHEN YOU CAN'T GET TO SLEEP

If you find yourself lying awake after zero hour and not feeling sleepy at all, follow the same process as above. It may be that your body clock is not ready for sleep, so sit and read or listen to the radio until you do feel sleepy.

The important thing is that it doesn't become a source of anxiety. It might take a few weeks to figure out your ideal sleep schedule—the time that suits you best to go to sleep and the optimum amount of sleep you need. Remember, everybody is different. See it as an experiment and, rather than worrying that you can't get to sleep, take an interest in the way you are feeling and see how it changes from night to night.

You might want to keep a sleep diary, with notes on how successful you were in getting to sleep, how tired you felt when you went to bed and when you woke up, whether you woke up during the night and what was on your mind. By writing it all down, you can see how things change over time and how the adjustments you make affect your state of mind. It also helps make it an interesting experiment rather than a source of annoyance and worry.

Keep a positive mindset as you adjust to your new routine and you will adjust more readily.

ENJOY BREAKING FREE

You're ready to kill the Little Monster and remove any last obstacles to a good night's sleep. Remember, you have nothing to sacrifice, only wonderful gains to make. Any fear you might feel is just last-minute nerves, like a skydiver about to jump. You know you've prepared everything perfectly and that the jump will feel exhilarating. You are the lucky fly on the wall of the pitcher plant that is being given the power to fly away. Take it!

Remind yourself of all the things you stand to gain:

Energy
Good health
More balanced moods
Better relationships
Higher self-esteem
Less stress
Better concentration
Clearer thinking
Happiness

All because you have regained control over your life.

When you recognize all the benefits of your new lifestyle choices, killing the Little Monster becomes a source of genuine pleasure, rather than something to dread, as so many people implementing change (including addicts) do. Let's examine the process in more detail and allay any lingering concerns you may have.

Chapter 17

KILLING THE LITTLE MONSTER

•CALM CONSCIOUSNESS •THOSE "TERRIBLE" SYMPTOMS
•WITHDRAWAL WITH WILLPOWER •DEATH THROES
•AFTERMATH

You've destroyed the Big Monster, you know you want to quit those sleep-disruptive foods, drinks, drugs, and lifestyle choices you've identified, and you understand all the arguments for doing so. Still, you might have a lingering fear that it's not going to be as easy as we have been telling you all along.

There is a common misconception that coming off any addictive drug means going through an unpleasant withdrawal period. The theory goes that as the toxins leave your body, you suffer a severe physical reaction. Typical symptoms include headaches, upset stomach, weak and aching muscles, heart palpitations, the shakes, the sweats, the shivers, and breathing difficulty.

Some people claim to have experienced such symptoms when quitting behavioral addictions, such as gambling or overspending, which don't involve putting poison into your body. So it can't be anything physical, can it? It has to be mental.

As with all the other excuses addicts give for not stopping, withdrawal pain is a myth. However, the theory is widely supported by so-called experts within the medical profession and the belief that it is true is enough to keep a lot of people from even trying to quit.

We have talked about the restless feeling you get as the effects of your fix wear off. It's the same for gambling, overspending, or sugar addiction as it is for nicotine and alcohol. The Little Monster cries out for more, creating a feeling of mild discomfort. That feeling is so slight as to be almost imperceptible. Addicts put up with it every day, largely without being conscious of it. It's only when they are prevented from having their next fix that it becomes a problem.

Promise a child a candy bar and they will become fixated on that thought until they get it. Delay the delivery of the candy bar and the child will become very restless and bad-tempered. As adults, we are affected in the same way, but we can make sure we get our fix when we want it, so we rarely make ourselves go without.

Let's say you're driving down the highway and you decide to stop for a cup of coffee and a snack at the next gas station. You start looking forward to it immediately. When you get there, however, the gas station is closed, so you have to drive to the next one. It's 10 miles down the road. All the way, you will be itching for that cup of coffee and that snack.

And that is about the extent of it—an itch. That's how "severe" the physical effect of withdrawal really is, but it's still enough to dominate your thoughts and behavior until you satisfy the craving. It's the Big Monster that makes withdrawal feel hard. The cries of the Little Monster are so faint that most addicts aren't even conscious of them—they trigger the Big Monster and those mental cravings.

Perhaps you have assumed that there's something different about the withdrawal you go through when you quit for good.

There isn't.

For most addicts who quit, there are none of the abnormal physical symptoms described above: no sweats or shakes, no headaches or palpitations. There are millions of addicts whose sleep has yet to become disrupted—they manage to go for hours every night without their fix, and the physical effects don't wake them up.

Now, if you were to stand in the way of them having that first fix the next day, they might react as if you'd stomped on their toe. But that's not a reaction to physical pain; it's panic at the prospect of being deprived. Once they are confident again of knowing that the next fix is coming, this panic subsides. If it were a physical pain, like a toothache, it would be there all the time. The craving the Big Monster causes is a real physical feeling—with no physical cause. It's created by thoughts. The great news is that we can change our thoughts in a heartbeat.

CALM CONSCIOUSNESS

You have probably experienced the panic feeling yourself. Most addicts have, whatever their addiction. It's the panic that sets in when you don't know where your next fix is coming from. Drinkers and smokers will go to great lengths to make sure they have a stock of booze or cigarettes so they know they're not going to be denied.

Sneaking out of the house, lying about where you're going, borrowing money from strangers, even putting yourself in dangerous situations—it's all common behavior among addicts, designed to avoid the panic feeling.

You do occasionally meet an addict who claims not to know the panic feeling. They vehemently claim never to have experienced the panic of not knowing where their next fix is going to come from. It doesn't take much probing to find out why: they are so afraid of finding themselves in that position that they take every precaution to make sure it never happens!

Every addict who is denied the opportunity to get their fix when they expect to experiences the panic feeling, and this is the real cause of any unpleasant withdrawal symptoms you might have heard about when people quit.

THOSE "TERRIBLE" SYMPTOMS

Let's look at those symptoms again:

Tiredness

Headaches

Upset stomach

Weak and aching muscles

Heart palpitations

The shakes

The sweats

The shivers

Difficulty breathing

They are just like flu symptoms, aren't they? In fact, some people describe withdrawal as being like a mild flu. The flu is horrible, and it can be very serious. But do you fear getting a mild case of the flu? You probably have already, several times in your life. Does the thought that you might get it again make you panic? Even if it did, wouldn't you be prepared to withstand a few days of the flu for a lifetime of freedom from insomnia?

We actually have a powerful resilience to pain. Pain only induces panic when you are not in control of it. Try pinching yourself and see how much you can endure before you have to stop. Now imagine it is someone else pinching you, and think about how you would react. It's panic that makes us react long before we reach the limit of endurance.

If you go to the gym or an exercise class, you know that it can be painful when you really push yourself, but the feeling doesn't make you panic. You actually enjoy it because you know that you control it—plus, it's an indication that you are doing something good for yourself.

Pain is not the problem here; the physical symptoms listed above are brought on by the fear and panic that pain induces if you don't understand why you're feeling it or what the consequences might be. It doesn't have to be a strong pain; it can be a mild discomfort. If you don't understand what's causing it, it can induce fear.

Take the mental reaction out of the picture and the symptoms of withdrawal are nothing more than a slight restlessness, like an itch wanting to be scratched. Watch nicotine addicts when they are denied the opportunity to smoke or vape. They will be restless and fidgety. You will notice little nervous tics, and they will constantly be doing things with their hands or grinding their teeth.

This restlessness is triggered by the empty, insecure feeling of withdrawal. It's not enough to even wake them up at night. But it can quickly turn into frustration, irritability, anxiety, anger, fear, and panic if they are not able to satisfy their craving.

It should be pretty clear now that addiction is the cause of this feeling, and continuing to feed the Little Monster does not relieve it. As long as you understand that, you will be in control and you will have no fear or panic when you quit.

Continue to feed the Little Monster and you will suffer from the restlessness for the rest of your life.

WITHDRAWAL WITH WILLPOWER

It is the fear of being deprived that turns this slight restlessness into panic. Once you've destroyed the Big Monster, there is no feeling of being deprived when you can't get your fix, and the feeble cries of the Little Monster are just that—feeble.

But if you still believe you're being deprived when you try to kill the Little Monster—as is the case with the willpower method—the withdrawal pangs will induce fear and panic, and you will suffer both physically and mentally.

Imagine having a permanent itch that you're not allowed to scratch; in addition, you believe the itch will last for the rest of your life unless you're allowed to scratch it. How long do you think you could last before your willpower gave in and you scratched the itch? If you did manage to hold out for a week or even more, imagine the relief you would feel when you finally gave in.

This is a description of the torture that addicts go through when trying to quit with the willpower method. It's the Big Monster that gives you the urge to scratch the itch. Destroy the Big Monster and you can live with it quite happily until it disappears completely.

The problem for addicts who quit with the willpower method is that, for them, the urge to scratch the itch does not die with the Little Monster. The Big Monster lives on and is triggered by everything they ever associated with their fix, such as unwinding after a day's work, seeing friends, and going to parties. Smokers, for example, think, "I used to smoke on these occasions," and they still believe they're being deprived.

The belief that the fix provides some sort of pleasure or crutch is a figment of the addict's imagination, left over from the brainwashing. The word "fix" came into use because addicts believe it fixes them. It certainly does that —not in the way they think, but in a far more sinister sense.

It's like applying ointment to a sore in the belief that it will clear it up, when all it does is turn the sore into a rash. If you were in that situation and were told all you had to do was leave the sore for a few days and it would heal on its own, you'd have no need or desire for the ointment.

It's easy to kick your addictions when you realize that the empty, insecure feeling of wanting a fix is caused by the last fix you had, and that the one thing that will make you suffer from that feeling for the rest of your life would be to have another. And it's easy to change your sleep-disruptive diet and behaviors when you know that the ones you adopted in the past fooled you into thinking they were beneficial when, of course, they were not. The combination of sleep-disruptive addiction, behavior, and lifestyle choices almost destroyed you—this is the wonderful moment where you can walk free, confident of great sleep.

When this is clear in your mind, you will endure none of the suffering you might have experienced in previous attempts to change because you will no longer believe you're being deprived of anything beneficial. On the contrary, you will experience a wonderful sense of freedom.

DEATH THROES

After implementing your list of changes and a new timetable, you might experience a slight craving for a few days. This is not a physical pain; it's just the faint cries of the Little Monster wanting to be fed. It wants you to either provide it with another fix of a drug you've escaped from or return to old, sleep-disruptive behavior. Before, it would have been the subconscious trigger for you to have your next fix, or eat junk, or forgo exercise etc. Now, you don't need to respond to it at all.

Nor do you need to close your mind to the feeling, though. The more you try not to think about it, the more it will remain at the front of your mind. If you are told not to think about elephants, what is the first thing you think of?

Elephants.

Feel free to use the faint cries of the Little Monster as a reminder of the wonderful gains you are making. Keep in mind that the Little Monster was created when you first started your sleep-disruptive behavior or addiction, and it has continued to feed on every subsequent fix or response to it . As soon as you stop, you simply cut off the supply, and that evil Little Monster begins to die.

In its death throes, the Little Monster will try to entice you to feed it. It may nag for a while, but you can still take pleasure in it by using that nagging feeling to create a mental image of this parasite getting weaker and weaker, and enjoy starving it to death.

Be ruthless. Take pleasure in feeling the Little Monster die. Even if you do get that feeling of "I need a fix" for a few days, don't worry about it. It's just the Little Monster doing everything it can to tempt you to feed it. As long as you're prepared for that, you will find it easy to keep starving it. You now have complete control over it. It's no longer destroying you; you are destroying it, and soon you will be free of it forever.

AFTERMATH

While the Little Monster is dying, you don't need to stand by and wait. You can keep enjoying the genuine pleasure of your new life from the moment you stop feeding it. That is the moment you choose to be free. There is nothing more to wait for.

Unlike addicts who quit with the willpower method, you don't have to torture yourself waiting for something to <u>not</u> happen.

For most people it takes just a few days for the Little Monster to die. That's a few days before the craving disappears altogether. During these few days, people who use the willpower method tend to feel completely obsessed with fighting the temptation to relapse; but then, after about three weeks, they suddenly realize that it's been a while since they thought about it. It's an exciting feeling… and a dangerous one.

One moment, they believed that life would always be miserable without their little crutch; now, they are convinced that time will solve their problem. They feel on top of the world. It's time to celebrate. What possible harm could it do to reward themselves with just one fix? Don't do it. Keep smiling, enjoying your freedom from the substances or behavior and great sleep.

Don't allow that sense of success to cause you to drop your guard—it's a familiar pattern and a sure way of snatching defeat from the jaws of victory. Once you've established your new lifestyle, behavior, and diet, all of which will work to ensure you achieve great sleep, don't tinker with it and never take it for granted. Cherish it.

If you find that you struggle with any particular addiction, behavior, or appetite, then please don't lose heart. All the other changes you have made will certainly allow you to succeed. And if you would like some help to free yourself of any of the specific issues I've mentioned, please get in touch. Easyway has already been applied to smoking, vaping, alcohol, cocaine, cannabis, opioids, prescription drugs, sugar addiction/weight, emotional eating, debt, gambling, caffeine, mindfulness, and even fear of flying, with many more being added each year. Visit www. AllenCarr.com

I cannot stress this enough—with your list of changes and your new timetable—you are not building a fragile house of cards likely to collapse if you struggle or even fail with one item. Instead, you will succeed in achieving great sleep in spite of that, leaving you free to address that outstanding issue more specifically in due course.

Chapter 18

GETTING FREE

•*A GRADUAL AWAKENING* •*START AT THE BEGINNING*
•*LOOKING FORWARD TO SLEEP* •*WAKING UP HAPPY*

If you have followed all the instructions so far, you have created—or started to create—a lifestyle that is ideally suited to healthy sleep. You're all set to start doing regular exercise, eating a healthier diet without feeling that you are depriving yourself, drinking only in moderation (or not at all), not smoking or vaping or partaking of any other form of nicotine, nor taking any addictive drugs.

You are keeping your caffeine consumption to the mornings only, if at all, and allowing enough time in the evening to unwind before bedtime, prepare your plans for the following day, and get to sleep in peace and comfort for somewhere between seven and nine hours.

In your mind you have changed your impression of yourself from an insomniac to someone who had a sleep problem but is now dealing with it, and is on track to restoring your sleep/wake cycle to the healthy balance that you were born to enjoy.

You will regard bed as a luxurious haven, a place you look forward to being, that is both comfortable and secure and where you get your blissful beauty sleep night after night.

If you feel that any of the elements described above are not yet in place, you may need to go back and read some chapters again; but that is only if you have some lingering doubt about your ability to achieve these conditions.

There is no rush, no need to fret. The cure for your sleep problem is a natural transition that involves every aspect of your waking life. You may have a lot of changes to make, or you may just have one fundamental change that is going to make all the difference. As long as you stay positive, remove any doubts in your ability to resolve your sleep problem, and follow the instructions, you will succeed.

A GRADUAL AWAKENING

When I devised my method for quitting smoking, I built up to the moment when you smoke your final cigarette. That is the moment that you fly away from the trap and begin the rest of your life as a happy non-smoker.

This moment has proven hugely symbolic in helping smokers quit. Some of them become so revolted by the idea of smoking as they are going through the method that they don't even want that final cigarette when the time comes. Others smoke their final cigarette down to the filter, unconvinced that they are going to break free. Others feel great joy at the final cigarette ritual. In any of those cases, they succeed. All I ask them to do is take pleasure in stubbing out their final cigarette and making a solemn vow never to smoke again. It is a moment of finality. Although the Little Monster has yet to die, the Big Monster is well and truly dead and the prison door is wide open. Stepping through the door is a wonderful moment that people who quit with Easyway remember for the rest of their lives.

You may be wondering when you can enjoy that moment of finality. The fact is, you already have—when you killed the Big Monster.

The point is this: with smoking, it's important to have the final cigarette because the method requires you to stop completely and never smoke again. There is no gradual cutting down. Cutting down, like dieting, merely creates a sense of deprivation, which in turn puts a heightened value on the next fix and makes it harder to quit.

So, with addictive drugs like nicotine, it is essential that you stop feeding the Little Monster at once.

Lifestyle and many behavioral changes, however, need to happen more gradually. With eating, for example, you can't just stop. Eating is necessary to satisfy hunger, and when we do it normally, it is a source of genuine pleasure. Why would we want you to cut anything out of your life that gives you genuine pleasure? We wouldn't. That would defeat the purpose entirely. We want you to enjoy life to the full.

The transition you are making from miserable insomniac to happy sleeper happens over a period of time, but that doesn't mean there is no exhilarating "parachute jump" moment when you realize you have done it. That comes when you unravel the brainwashing and see things as they really are.

Once you've stopped the cycle of sleep disruption, you can enjoy building your new sleep-healthy lifestyle.

The ninth instruction is:

Take it gradually.

START AT THE BEGINNING

Ease yourself into your new routines. Apply the changes in timetable and behaviors, but only gradually change the types of food you eat and when you eat them. In the evenings, it's good to have a lighter meal. So experiment with avoiding refined sugar and processed and starchy carbs in the evenings. Rather than make meat the main focus of your meal, either cut it out altogether or have it as a smaller side dish, so that the majority of your plate is made up of fresh salad and vegetables. Avoid heavy dressings and learn to enjoy fresh flavors again; it's amazing how quickly you rediscover your natural tastes. It's an easy change to make because those are the foods that taste the best too. Once you get into the routine of eating them regularly, you will find that they become your favorites. It's remarkable. When you pay attention to your senses, you discover that the most nutritious food also happens to be the tastiest.

Of course, this is no coincidence. It's how we are designed. In fact, it's how all animals are designed—to find the most pleasure in the foods that are best for them. Why else would they eat those foods? Koalas don't have books on nutrition; they just know that they like eucalyptus leaves. Grass tastes good to cows. Lions like raw meat. Every creature is designed to love the food it needs most.

Take time to feel completely at ease with your first steps before you move on to bigger changes. Rush it and there is a danger that you will start feeling deprived. Impatience will cause unnecessary stress. A gradual transition is nothing to worry about. You need to give your body and mind time to adjust.

The beauty is that there is no need to feel impatient, because you have already sprung the trap. You have achieved the mindset change that we set out to achieve at the beginning of the book, and all that remains is for the change to gather momentum.

You have your mind set on making lifestyle changes that will have a profound effect on your health and happiness. Any change can be unsettling, even when it is as obviously beneficial as this is. If you take it too fast, you could actually make it slower. The saying "more haste, less speed" certainly applies in this case.

Soon, the small changes you make as your first steps will become second nature (we should really say first nature, since this is the lifestyle nature designed for you). As you rediscover the pleasure of eating the tastiest foods, putting energy into your body, enjoying natural exercise (even if it's just incorporating a brisk walk into your morning and afternoon routine), freeing your mind from stress and anxiety before bedtime and giving yourself a chance to fully rest and recuperate, you will wonder why you ever lived any other way.

As you begin to feel those benefits, as sleep starts to come more easily and you feel more awake during the day, you will realize that the method is working. And because it is this easy, you will feel confident that it will keep working. You might even explore other changes that you perhaps resisted initially.

Changing what you eat in the evening alone is enough to make a difference. It is the spark that will start a chain reaction, reversing the vicious circles we described in Chapter 3 and turning them into virtuous circles, where benefit leads to pleasure, which drives the pursuit of the benefit, and so on.

LOOKING FORWARD TO SLEEP

The greatest virtuous circle of all is the sleep cycle. Good sleep restores your body and cleanses the mind, leading to greater health and vigor, resulting in less stress and anxiety and a better diet, aiding better sleep.

Insomnia is a source of stress and anxiety in itself. You begin to dread night-time, knowing that it's just going to be another bout of restlessness and a mental wrestling match, leaving you feeling tired and irritable in the morning.

As you begin to apply your new sleep routine, however, along with your lifestyle changes, you attack the vicious circle of insomnia at multiple points. You give yourself a chance at a better night's sleep. You put less strain on your body and mind so they require less restorative sleep. You build your health and vigor through diet and exercise. You reduce your exposure to stress and anxiety and remove the desire for junk food, drugs, and other addictive behaviors.

That destructive cycle grinds to a halt and a much healthier, happy cycle takes its place. This is the natural cycle that all creatures are designed to go through when they sleep. It is the natural cycle that you were born to follow. It is effortless and self-

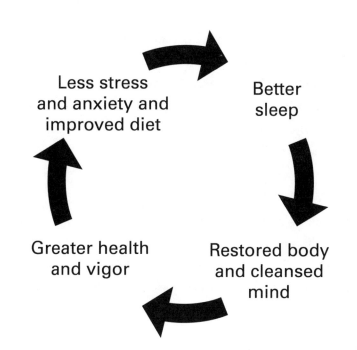

perpetuating. Once you get it turning again, it will run itself, as long as you continue to follow your routine.

You will be happy to do so because it is a wonderful routine—one that gives you the bliss of a good night's sleep and brings you health, vigor, and happiness in the daytime. You will look back on the time when you feared that the changes you needed to make would leave you feeling miserable about life and wonder what on earth you were thinking.

Now, at any time of day, you can look forward to sleep with the same joy that you would look forward to coming home to a loved one. That doesn't mean you should crave your bed all day long. The consequence of healthy sleep is increased energy while you are awake. It's just that the thought of bedtime will fill you with joy and confidence, not the dread you used to feel.

You can begin to look forward to sleep in this way from the moment you begin your new sleep routine. While it might take time to fully reverse the cycle, you will begin to notice improvements right away. That's the sign that the method is working; the vicious circle is grinding to a halt and soon the virtuous circle will be purring into action.

Imagine how that will feel. Rather than dreading going to bed at night, you can look forward to sleep with nothing but joy, knowing that the fear of a lifetime of insomnia is behind you and you never again have to worry about losing sleep, nor the effect it has on your health.

It's a wonderful feeling. Until you restore the healthy sleep cycle, you cannot fully gauge how heavily sleep loss affects you, both physically and mentally. It is a crushing pressure that builds over time and slowly squeezes the life out of you. You know it's not a good feeling, and you stress about how it is affecting you. But all the while you believe you can keep living the way you do and hope that one day it will resolve itself.

But bad lifestyle choices do not resolve themselves. On the contrary, they become increasingly destructive until you do something positive to change them.

It's only when you reverse the vicious circle and feel the cycle turning in your favor that you realize what a burden sleep loss really is. The cumulative benefits of improving all those points in the circle give you a lightness and ease of spirit that feel like emerging into the light from under a dark, heavy cloud.

Looking back at the natural warning signs in Chapter 13, take note of the changes:

Whereas before you were negative and moody, now you take a positive approach and are upbeat about new ideas and suggestions.

Whereas before you were often irritable, now you are full of joy and ready to share it with others.

Whereas before you had difficulty concentrating, now you approach your work with focus and interest.

Whereas before you craved junk food as a source of comfort, now you look forward to eating healthy food and the cravings are becoming rarer.

Whereas before you felt constant anxiety, now your worries are much less frequent and you can trace them back to real issues, which you can deal with.

WAKING UP HAPPY

When you suffer from a sleep disorder, waking up in the morning is often accompanied by anxious thoughts. "What time is it?" "I didn't sleep again." "I'm exhausted." "I've got so much to do."

As you adjust to your new lifestyle, you might find that anxious thoughts are still with you first thing in the morning, and that might lead you to think you have not solved your sleep problem at all. That is not the case. You can get into a habit of having anxious thoughts when you wake up, even after a good night's sleep, but it's a habit you can break with practice.

Just as you need to be ready for the death throes of the Little Monster, you need to be ready for those moments when you wake up with a start. Remember, you made your plans for the day last night, so there is nothing you have overlooked that is going to bite you.

Prepare your positive thoughts. Think about what makes you genuinely happy and, as soon as you wake up, go there in your mind. Picture yourself doing the things you enjoy most. You can prepare these thoughts at any time of day so that you have them ready when you wake up.

If anxious thoughts barge in, let them pass, and bring your mind back to the happy thoughts. Some people find that it helps to list three things for which you are grateful, and think about those things.

This all helps release your mind from anxious thoughts and steer it onto positive, happy thoughts. After a while, this will become your default mindset when you wake up. No more perceived threats that don't really exist. Just relaxed, confident thoughts.

While you are practicing your morning meditation, make sure you are in a comfortable position, ideally on your back, breathing steadily in through your nose and out through your mouth. This will help your body relax, which in turn will help your mind relax.

Do not look at your phone or other devices. If you've followed our advice, they should be out of reach in another room anyway. As soon as you turn on your device and go online, you open a gate for all the world and its problems to flood into your mind. If you have to look, save it for later.

If you wake up to an alarm clock, try to find one that is not too jarring when it goes off. Sure, the idea of an alarm clock is to wake you up, but not to wake you up thinking the house is on fire! You want to wake up gently, not with your heart pounding and adrenaline flooding through your veins.

Just as you have prepared your pre-sleep routine, prepare a morning routine too—one that you always look forward to. Avoid lying in bed too long after you've woken up. Chatting with your partner is great, but after a while it's good to get up and start your day. Your morning routine can include a refreshing shower, a delicious breakfast, and some light exercise that is not so demanding that you dread having to do it, but vigorous enough to get your heart rate up and the endorphins flowing. Dancing to your favorite music is a great way to start your day and get your body going.

The more you have prepared the night before, the more relaxed your mornings will be. And the more relaxed your mornings are, the more you will look forward to sleep at night. So as well as planning tomorrow's tasks during your wind-down to bedtime, put out the clothes you want to wear, check what the weather is going to be like, set the table for breakfast, and do anything else you can do that will make your morning easy.

Mornings can be very stressful times, especially if you have young children. But you can take away that stress by preparing in advance. With conscious preparation, you can turn mornings into wonderful times, when you look forward to a new day with all the potential for happiness and fulfillment that it brings, and embrace that potential with renewed energy and enthusiasm.

Chapter 19

THE PURSUIT
OF HAPPINESS

•BROKEN NIGHTS •HEALTH AND FITNESS
•A BALANCED LIFE •THE TWO WOODCUTTERS

In Chapter 4, we quoted Thomas Jefferson's statement in the Declaration of Independence, that the pursuit of happiness is every person's "unalienable right." The pursuit of happiness is exactly what this book is about. It is what Easyway is about.

I was once a heavy smoker who had tried everything to quit but failed time after time. Each failure made me more and more miserable. I was resigned to a life of slavery and dying a nasty, miserable death. I could see the end, but could do nothing to prevent it—until I discovered the simple truth:

Quitting does not have to be hard.

In fact, you are more likely to succeed if you follow a method that makes it easy. After discovering this truth, I started spreading the word and bringing the same joy I had discovered to millions of other addicts. The pursuit of happiness lay behind everything I did.

We could go into detail about all the medical impacts of sleep deprivation and quote the research that has gone into understanding why it happens and what scientists think can be done about it. But it can be much more easily summed up in one phrase: sleep deprivation makes you unhappy.

Unhappiness is a clear signal from the Incredible Machine that something is wrong. It is a signal we are supposed to respond to, just as you would respond if a doctor told you that you had a life-threatening illness and needed to change some aspects of your lifestyle in order to avoid disaster. You have responded by picking up this book and reading it all the way to the end.

To repeat what I said at the beginning of Chapter 16, if you haven't read the book all the way to this point, if you have just skipped to the end hoping to find the magic formula for curing your sleep problem, I'm very sorry, but it does not work that way.

Easyway is not magic; it is a carefully thought-out method based on first-hand experience and a deep understanding of the psychological struggles than can affect the mind of anybody. It is a method that needs to be followed from start to finish. Skip any part and it's like skipping one digit of the combination to a safe. The door will remain firmly locked.

If you have read the whole book up to this point, congratulations! You have the complete combination to unlock the door, and all you need to do is use it.

The tenth instruction is:

Open the prison door and start enjoying life to the full!

The pursuit of happiness begins in bed. You can smile at that, but it's true. Whichever way you look at it, bed is a place where all the ingredients for happiness are supposed to come together: pleasure, contentment, satisfaction, fulfillment, peace, and health.

Any doubts you had about having the necessary willpower or even being capable of curing your sleep problems are now buried in the past. Any fears that changing your lifestyle would be hard and miserable are now far from your mind as you grow accustomed to the new, sleep-friendly life you are living and all the benefits it brings.

Let's face it, nothing drastic has changed. You are still the same person you were when you first picked up this book. To all intents and purposes, you are living the same life, just with a few small adjustments that make a big difference. You have not had to give up anything. All that has gone from your life is the fog of illusions that had conned you into a situation where you felt stressed and anxious and, ultimately, were losing sleep.

Those illusions were built up over your whole lifetime to date. It took the time it takes to read this book to blow them away.

BROKEN NIGHTS

Curing a chronic sleep problem does not mean you will never have another broken night. There will be nights when you can't get to sleep or you are woken and lie awake for hours. But now you have a strategy for dealing with that. Importantly, these nights will be the exception, not the norm. Doesn't that in itself sound fabulous?

We are not pretending that, if you've followed the method all the way, your life will be one of permanent bliss. We all know life is not like that—and we wouldn't want it to be. The hard times make the good times better.

There will be worries, there will be stress, there may even be times when you drink more than you know you should, or spend too much time on social media, or your Junk Margin starts to get a bit large. But you don't need to panic. You know what to do and you understand what's going on.

It doesn't mean that everything you have learned and the changes you have made are all a waste of time. You're not going to be fooled by those illusions again because once you have seen through an illusion you can never be fooled by it again.

So remain calm, pay attention to what your body is telling you, go back to your pre-sleep routine, check your diet and exercise routine, and see if you can identify what is out of balance. You know what you are looking for now, and you know how to look.

Whatever is happening in your life, put sleep front and center of your recovery plan.

HEALTH AND FITNESS

Your body is an Incredible Machine capable of performing a multitude of tasks at the same time. Rejoice in the fact that you have this living, breathing machine and take pride in taking care of it.

All it asks is that you put the right kind of fuel in when it needs it. Do that and the on-board computer will take care of everything else. It will tell you when the machine is fired up and raring to go, and it will tell you when the machine needs to rest. As long as you respond to the signals, it will reward you with natural hormones that create the emotion in your brain that we know as happiness.

Eat well, exercise regularly, respond when you feel pain or discomfort. Treat yourself kindly. After all, this is not just any machine we are talking about; this is YOU!

When you hear the words "health and fitness," you might have a vision of an athlete or a personal trainer or one of those people who likes to go out running, and you might be thinking, "That's just not me." That is not a problem. You just need to keep your body in good health and exercise at a level that you find comfortable and enjoyable. It's even better if you can fit it into your normal day—for example, by getting on or off the bus a 30-minute walk from your destination rather than at the closest stop.

Of course, you are not going to be able to exercise as hard at the age of 80 as you did when you were 20. But no one is asking you to. As long as you pay attention to your fuel gauge and get the fuel you need to match the energy you burn, your body will remain in balance.

How will you know? Because your body will tell you.

If you enjoyed sports in the past and have simply been out of the routine of engaging with them—go for it. As long as you're enjoying it, it all adds to your sleep-friendly lifestyle.

A BALANCED LIFE

When you get everything in balance—intake and output, activity and sleep, work and play—life feels easy. It's like having a finely tuned car. You don't think about what's going on under the hood, you just enjoy driving it. Your mind is free to think about other things: positive, creative things, things that make you happy.

It becomes self-perpetuating. The virtuous circle feeds itself.

Remember the elements of that virtuous circle and check on them every so often, just to make sure you are keeping everything in balance. It doesn't require much thought. You certainly don't need to stress about it. Just remember the importance of sleep, diet, and exercise in keeping that cycle going and keep in mind that if any one of those elements becomes deficient, the other two will be affected.

In focusing on a balanced diet and a balanced sleep/wake cycle, be careful not to overlook the balance between work and play. Some people say they want to learn how to sleep better just so they can keep flogging themselves to death with work. They need the extra energy so they can work longer hours.

It's a clear sign that there is something wrong. Flogging yourself into the ground will not make you sleep better; it will make you sleep worse, because it throws everything out of balance. Diet, routine, exercise, happiness—they all go out the window.

Moreover, it is not the way to improve your productivity. Keep flogging yourself and your energy, creative thinking, concentration, powers of organization, problem-solving ability and any other skills you need to apply for work will diminish at an increasing rate. You will slow down, you will make mistakes, and you will upset people and get upset yourself.

You've achieved something wonderful. Allow yourself to

feel good about it. Take care of yourself and remember, the more sleep-friendly lifestyle choices, food, and drink you adopt, and the more sleep-disruptive food, drink, and drugs you avoid, the better you will feel.

In order to have all your faculties functioning at full power, you need to balance work with rest. Getting all the rest your need doesn't mean you are lazy or work-shy. On the contrary, it shows that you take the trouble to maintain the Incredible Machine to operate at full power. And the better the machine operates, the less you have to strain yourself.

To illustrate the point, let's end with a story. It seems appropriate.

THE TWO WOODCUTTERS

There were two woodcutters called Sam and Dan. They were always arguing about who could chop the most wood, so they decided to have a competition. Starting at dawn, they would chop wood until dusk and then see who had chopped the most.

The next morning they got to it. After a while, Dan paused for breath and glanced over at Sam, who was sitting against a tree. "Ha!" thought Dan. "Tired already. I've got this in the bag."An hour later, the same thing happened. Dan stopped chopping and glanced over at Sam, who was sitting once again against a tree. "This is easy," thought Dan, who kept chopping away.

So it went for the rest of the day, with the same pattern repeating itself every hour or so, and when the sun set Dan couldn't wait to claim victory. To Dan's amazement, though, Sam had chopped the most wood. There was no disputing it. Sam's pile was much bigger than Dan's.

"How did you do it?" cried Dan. "Every time I looked over at you, you were sitting with your back against a tree!" "It's simple," said Sam. "Every time you saw me resting, while you kept chopping, I was sharpening my ax." Sweet dreams!

Chapter 20

REFERENCE

THE INSTRUCTIONS

If, from time to time, you need a quick reminder of the method and what you have learned along the way, keep this book handy. For easy reference, here is a reminder of the instructions. It's good to take a look at them every now and then, just to reinforce your newfound strength.

We have shown which chapter they are in, in case you want to go back and read any part again.

1. Follow ALL the instructions in order. (Ch1)

2. Keep an open mind. (Ch1)

3. Reject anything that goes against Mother Nature's guide. (Ch2)

4. Begin with a feeling of elation. (Ch4)

5. Question everything you think you know about sleep, addiction, and behaviors. (Ch6)

6. Never doubt your decision to change. (Ch9)

7. Ignore any advice that conflicts with Easyway. (Ch10)

8. Exercise only for pleasure. (Ch14)

9. Take it gradually. (Ch18)

10. Open the prison door and start enjoying life to the full! (Ch19)

YOUR NEW SLEEP ROUTINE

Zero hour
The time you need to be falling asleep.

Zero minus 30
Begin your wind-down.

Take a hot bath or shower and go to bed with a book or something soothing on the radio. Alternatively, lie in bed and meditate. The important thing is that you are not doing anything stimulating or agitating.

Set the bedroom temperature no higher than 64°F. Go to the bathroom.

Place a glass of water by the bed in case you wake up feeling thirsty.

Make sure you are truly comfortable in bed.

When you're ready, turn out the light. Practice steady breathing, in through the nose, out through the mouth, and allow your mind to relax and drift off to sleep.

Zero minus 1 hour

Switch off all digital devices and remove them from your bedroom.

Look ahead to tomorrow and write down any tasks or concerns that are making you feel anxious. Plan how you are going to tackle those tasks and concerns the next day.

Zero minus 3 hours

Try to be done with your evening meal. Try to avoid eating after this time, and definitely don't drink alcohol.

If you prefer to exercise in the evening, you have the next two hours in which to do so.

Zero minus 12 hours

Avoid any caffeine after this time.

Zero minus 16 hours

Wake-up time. Try to get out of bed as soon as possible and start your day.

Eat a healthy breakfast, preferably one with plenty of fruit and a few nuts and seeds.

If you prefer to exercise in the morning, build it into this time.

EPILOGUE

You've done an amazing thing – enjoy! Don't forget, if you ever have any questions or concerns about sleep or any other behavior or addiction issue, we'll be delighted to hear from you and happy to provide you with free-of-charge advice.

Visit www.AllenCarr.com or join our "Allen Carr's Easyway to Better Sleep" Facebook group.

ALLEN CARR'S EASYWAY CENTERS

The following list indicates the countries where Allen Carr's Easyway To Stop Smoking Centers are currently operational.

Check www.AllenCarr.com for latest additions to this list.

The success rate at the centers, based on the three-month money-back guarantee, is over 90 percent.

Selected centers also offer sessions that deal with alcohol, other drugs, and weight issues. Please check with your nearest center, listed on the following pages, for details.

Allen Carr's Easyway guarantee that you will find it easy to stop at the centers or your money back.

JOIN US!

Allen Carr's Easyway Centers have spread throughout the world with incredible speed and success. Our global franchise network now covers more than 150 cities in over 45 countries. This amazing growth has been achieved entirely organically. Former addicts, just like you, were so impressed by the ease with which they stopped that they felt inspired to contact us to see how they could bring the method to their region.

If you feel the same, contact us for details on how to become an Allen Carr's Easyway To Stop Smoking or an Allen Carr's Easyway To Stop Drinking franchisee.

Email us at: join-us@allencarr.com including your full name, postal address, and region of interest.

SUPPORT US!

No, don't send us money!

You have achieved something really marvelous. Every time we hear of someone escaping from the sinking ship, we get a feeling of enormous satisfaction.

It would give us great pleasure to hear that you have freed yourself from the slavery of addiction, so please visit the following web page where you can tell us of your success, inspire others to follow in your footsteps, and hear about ways you can help to spread the word.

 www.allencarr.com/fanzone

You can "like" our Facebook page here **www.facebook.com/ AllenCarr**

Together, we can help further Allen Carr's mission: to cure the world of addiction.

ALLEN CARR'S EASYWAY CENTERS

LONDON CLINIC AND WORLDWIDE HEAD OFFICE
Park House, 14 Pepys Road, Raynes Park, London SW20 8NH
Tel: +44 (0)20 8944 7761
Fax: +44 (0)20 8944 8619
Email: mail@allencarr.com
Website: www.allencarr.com
Therapists: John Dicey, Colleen Dwyer, Crispin Hay, Emma Hudson, Rob Fielding, Sam Kelser, Rob Groves, Debbie Brewer-West, Mark Keen, Duncan Bhaskaran-Brown, Mark Newman, Gerry Williams (Alcohol), Monique Douglas (Weight)

WORLDWIDE PRESS OFFICE
Tel: +44 (0)7970 88 44 52
Contact: John Dicey
Tel: +44 (0)7970 88 44 52
Email: media@allencarr.com

NORTH AMERICAN CENTERS

U.S.A.
Sessions held throughout the USA
Tel: +1 855 440 3777
Email: support@usa.allencarr.com
Website: www.allencarr.com

New York
Tel: +1 855 440 3777
Therapists: Natalie Clays and Team
Email: support@usa.allencarr.com
Website: www.allencarr.com

Los Angeles
Tel: +1 855 440 3777
Therapists: Natalie Clays and Team
Email: support@usa.allencarr.com
Website: www.allencarr.com

Milwaukee (and South Wisconsin)
Tel: +1 262 770 1260
Therapist: Wayne Spaulding
Email: wayne@easywaywisconsin.com
Website: www.allencarr.com

CANADA
Tel: +1 855 440 3777
Therapist: Natalie Clays
Email: natalie@ca.allencarr.com
Website: www.allencarr.com

U.K. CENTERS

UK Clinic Information and Central Booking Line

Tel: 0800 389 2115 (UK only)

Birmingham

Tel & Fax: 0800 389 2115
Therapists: John Dicey, Colleen Dwyer, Crispin Hay, Emma Hudson, Rob Fielding, Sam Kelser, Rob Groves, Debbie Brewer-West, Mark Keen, Duncan Bhaskaran-Brown, Mark Newman
Email: mail@allencarr.com
Website: www.allencarr.com

Bournemouth

Tel: 0800 389 2115
Therapists: John Dicey, Colleen Dwyer, Crispin Hay, Emma Hudson, Rob Fielding, Sam Kelser, Rob Groves, Debbie Brewer-West, Mark Keen, Duncan Bhaskaran-Brown, Mark Newman
Email: mail@allencarr.com
Website: www.allencarr.com

Brentwood

Tel: 0800 389 2115
Therapists: John Dicey, Colleen Dwyer, Crispin Hay, Emma Hudson, Rob Fielding, Sam Kelser, Rob Groves, Debbie Brewer-West, Mark Keen, Duncan Bhaskaran-Brown, Mark Newman
Email: mail@allencarr.com
Website: www.allencarr.com

Brighton

Tel: 0800 389 2115
Therapists: John Dicey, Colleen Dwyer, Crispin Hay, Emma Hudson, Rob Fielding, Sam Kelser, Rob Groves, Debbie Brewer-West, Mark Keen, Duncan Bhaskaran-Brown, Mark Newman
Email: mail@allencarr.com
Website: www.allencarr.com

Bristol

Tel: 0800 389 2115
Therapists: John Dicey, Colleen Dwyer, Crispin Hay, Emma Hudson, Rob Fielding, Sam Kelser, Rob Groves, Debbie Brewer-West, Mark Keen, Duncan Bhaskaran-Brown, Mark Newman
Email: mail@allencarr.com
Website: www.allencarr.com

Cambridge

Tel: 0800 389 2115
Therapists: John Dicey, Colleen Dwyer, Crispin Hay, Emma Hudson, Rob Fielding, Sam Kelser, Rob Groves, Debbie Brewer-West, Mark Keen, Duncan Bhaskaran-Brown, Mark Newman
Email: mail@allencarr.com
Website: www.allencarr.com

Coventry

Tel: 0800 321 3007
Therapist: Rob Fielding
Email: info@easywaymidlands.co.uk
Website: www.allencarr.com

Cumbria

Tel: 0800 389 2115
Therapists: John Dicey, Colleen
Dwyer, Crispin Hay, Emma
Hudson, Rob Fielding, Sam Kelser,
Rob Groves, Debbie Brewer-West,
Mark Keen, Duncan Bhaskaran-
Brown, Mark Newman
Email: mail@allencarr.com
Website: www.allencarr.com

Derby

Tel: 0800 389 2115
Therapists: John Dicey, Colleen
Dwyer, Crispin Hay, Emma
Hudson, Rob Fielding, Sam Kelser,
Rob Groves, Debbie Brewer-West,
Mark Keen, Duncan Bhaskaran-
Brown, Mark Newman
Email: mail@allencarr.com
Website: www.allencarr.com

Guernsey

Tel: 0800 077 6187
Therapist: Mark Keen
Email:
mark@easywaymanchester.co.uk
Website: www.allencarr.com

Isle of Man

Tel: 0800 077 6187
Therapist: Mark Keen
Email: mark@easywaymanchester.
co.uk
Website: www.allencarr.com

Jersey

Tel: 0800 077 6187
Therapist: Mark Keen
Email:
mark@easywaymanchester.co.uk
Website: www.allencarr.com

Kent

Tel: 0800 389 2115
Therapists: John Dicey, Colleen
Dwyer, Crispin Hay, Emma
Hudson, Rob Fielding, Sam Kelser,
Rob Groves, Debbie Brewer-West,
Mark Keen, Duncan Bhaskaran-
Brown, Mark Newman
Email: mail@allencarr.com
Website: www.allencarr.com

Lancashire

Tel: 0800 389 2115
Therapists: John Dicey, Colleen
Dwyer, Crispin Hay, Emma
Hudson, Rob Fielding, Sam Kelser,
Rob Groves, Debbie Brewer-West,
Mark Keen, Duncan Bhaskaran-
Brown, Mark Newman
Email: mail@allencarr.com
Website: www.allencarr.com

Leeds

Tel: 0800 077 6187
Therapist: Mark Keen
Email:
mark@easywaymanchester.co.uk
Website: www.allencarr.com

Leicester

Tel: 0800 321 3007
Therapist: Rob Fielding
Email:
info@easywaymidlands.co.uk
Website: www.allencarr.com

Lincoln

Tel: 0800 321 3007
Therapist: Rob Fielding
Email:
info@easywaymidlands.co.uk
Website: www.allencarr.com

Liverpool
Tel: 0800 389 2115
Therapists: John Dicey, Colleen
Dwyer, Crispin Hay, Emma
Hudson, Rob Fielding, Sam Kelser,
Rob Groves, Debbie Brewer-West,
Mark Keen, Duncan Bhaskaran-
Brown, Mark Newman
Email: mail@allencarr.com
Website: www.allencarr.com

Manchester
Tel: 0800 077 6187
Therapist: Mark Keen
Email:
mark@easywaymanchester.co.uk
Website: www.allencarr.com

Milton Keynes
Tel: 0800 389 2115
Therapists: John Dicey, Colleen
Dwyer, Crispin Hay, Emma
Hudson, Rob Fielding, Sam Kelser,
Rob Groves, Debbie Brewer-West,
Mark Keen, Duncan Bhaskaran-
Brown, Mark Newman
Email: mail@allencarr.com
Website: www.allencarr.com

Newcastle/North East
Tel: 0800 389 2115
Therapists: John Dicey, Colleen
Dwyer, Crispin Hay, Emma
Hudson, Rob Fielding, Sam Kelser,
Rob Groves, Debbie Brewer-West,
Mark Keen, Duncan Bhaskaran-
Brown, Mark Newman
Email:
mail@allencarr.com
Website: www.allencarr.com

Nottingham
Tel: 0800 389 2115
Therapists:John Dicey, Colleen
Dwyer, Crispin Hay, Emma
Hudson, Rob Fielding, Sam Kelser,
Rob Groves, Debbie Brewer-West,
Mark Keen, Duncan Bhaskaran-
Brown, Mark Newman
Email: mail@allencarr.com
Website: www.allencarr.com

Oxford
Tel: 0800 389 2115
Therapists: John Dicey, Colleen
Dwyer, Crispin Hay, Emma
Hudson, Rob Fielding, Sam Kelser,
Rob Groves, Debbie Brewer-West,
Mark Keen, Duncan Bhaskaran-
Brown, Mark Newman
Email: mail@allencarr.com
Website: www.allencarr.com

Reading
Tel: 0800 389 2115
Therapists: John Dicey, Colleen
Dwyer, Crispin Hay, Emma
Hudson, Rob Fielding, Sam Kelser,
Rob Groves, Debbie Brewer-West,
Mark Keen, Duncan Bhaskaran-
Brown, Mark Newman
Email: mail@allencarr.com
Website: www.allencarr.com

SCOTLAND
Glasgow and Edinburgh
Tel: +44 (0)131 449 7858
Therapists: Paul Melvin and Jim
McCreadie
Email: info@easywayscotland.co.uk
Website: www.allencarr.com

Southampton

Tel: 0800 389 2115
Therapists: John Dicey, Colleen
Dwyer, Crispin Hay, Emma
Hudson, Rob Fielding, Sam Kelser,
Rob Groves, Debbie Brewer-West,
Mark Keen, Duncan Bhaskaran-
Brown, Mark Newman
Email: mail@allencarr.com
Website: www.allencarr.com

Southport

Tel: 0800 389 2115
Therapists: John Dicey, Colleen
Dwyer, Crispin Hay, Emma
Hudson, Rob Fielding, Sam Kelser,
Rob Groves, Debbie Brewer-West,
Mark Keen, Duncan Bhaskaran-
Brown, Mark Newman
Email: mail@allencarr.com
Website: www.allencarr.com

Staines/Heathrow

Tel: 0800 389 2115
Therapists: John Dicey, Colleen
Dwyer, Crispin Hay, Emma
Hudson, Rob Fielding, Sam Kelser,
Rob Groves, Debbie Brewer-West,
Mark Keen, Duncan Bhaskaran-
Brown, Mark Newman
Email: mail@allencarr.com
Website: www.allencarr.com

Stevenage

Tel: 0800 389 2115
Therapists: John Dicey, Colleen
Dwyer, Crispin Hay, Emma
Hudson, Rob Fielding, Sam Kelser,
Rob Groves, Debbie Brewer-West,
Mark Keen, Duncan Bhaskaran-
Brown, Mark Newman
Email: mail@allencarr.com
Website: www.allencarr.com

Stoke

Tel: 0800 389 2115
Therapists: John Dicey, Colleen
Dwyer, Crispin Hay, Emma
Hudson, Rob Fielding, Sam Kelser,
Rob Groves, Debbie Brewer-West,
Mark Keen, Duncan Bhaskaran-
Brown, Mark Newman
Email: mail@allencarr.com
Website: www.allencarr.com

Surrey

Park House, 14 Pepys Road, Raynes
Park, London SW20 8NH
Tel: +44 (0)20 8944 7761
Fax: +44 (0)20 8944 8619
Therapists: John Dicey, Colleen
Dwyer, Crispin Hay, Emma
Hudson, Rob Fielding, Sam Kelser,
Rob Groves, Debbie Brewer-West,
Mark Keen, Duncan Bhaskaran-
Brown, Mark Newman
Gerry Williams (Alcohol), Monique
Douglas (Weight)
Email: mail@allencarr.com
Website: www.allencarr.com

Watford

Tel: 0800 389 2115
Therapists: John Dicey, Colleen
Dwyer, Crispin Hay, Emma
Hudson, Rob Fielding, Sam Kelser,
Rob Groves, Debbie Brewer-West,
Mark Keen, Duncan Bhaskaran-
Brown, Mark Newman
Email: mail@allencarr.com
Website: www.allencarr.com

Worcester

Tel: 0800 321 3007
Therapist: Rob Fielding
Email:
info@easywaymidlands.co.uk
Website: www.allencarr.com

WORLDWIDE CENTERS

AUSTRALIA
ACT, NSW, NT, QLD, VIC
Tel: 1300 848 028
Therapist: Natalie Clays and Team
Email: natalie@allencarr.com.au
Website: www.allencarr.com

South Australia
Tel: 1300 848 028
Therapist: Jaime Reed
Email: sa@allencarr.com.au
Website: www.allencarr.com

Western Australia
Tel: 1300 848 028
Therapist: Natalie Clays and Team
Email: natalie@allencarr.com.au
Website: www.allencarr.com

AUSTRIA
Sessions held throughout Austria
Freephone: 0800RAUCHEN
(0800 7282436)
Tel: +43 (0)3512 44755
Therapists: Erich Kellermann and
Team
Email: info@allen-carr.at
Website: www.allencarr.com

BELGIUM
Brussels
Tel: +32 (0)2 808 19 65
Therapist: Paula Rooduijn
Email: info@allencarr.be
Website: www.allencarr.com

BRAZIL
Therapist : Lilian Brunstein
Email:
contato@easywayonline.com.br
Website: www.allencarr.com

BULGARIA
Tel: 0800 14104 / +359 899 88 99 07
Therapist: Rumyana Kostadinova
Email: rk@nepushaveche.com
Website: www.allencarr.com

CHILE
Tel: +56 2 4744587
Therapist: Claudia Sarmiento
Email: contacto@allencarr.cl
Website: www.allencarr.com

CYPRUS
Tel: +357 25770611
Therapist: Andreas Damianou
Email: info@allencarr.com.cy
Website: www.allencarr.com

DENMARK
Sessions held throughout Denmark
Tel: +45 70267711
Therapist: Mette Fønss
Email: mette@easyway.dk
Website: www.allencarr.com

ESTONIA
Tel: +372 733 0044
Therapist: Henry Jakobson
Email: info@allencarr.ee
Website: www.allencarr.com

FINLAND
Tel: +358-(0)45 3544099
Therapist: Janne Ström
Email: info@allencarr.fi
Website: www.allencarr.com

FRANCE

Sessions held throughout France
Freephone: 0800 386387
Tel: +33 (4)91 33 54 55
Therapists: Erick Serre and Team
Email: info@allencarr.fr
Website: www.allencarr.com

GERMANY

Sessions held throughout Germany
Freephone: 08000RAUCHEN
(0800 07282436)
Tel: +49 (0)8031 90190-0
Therapists: Erich Kellermann
and Team
Email: info@allen-carr.de
Website: www.allencarr.com

GREECE

Sessions held throughout Greece
Tel: +30 210 5224087
Therapist: Panos Tzouras
Email: panos@allencarr.gr
Website: www.allencarr.com

GUATEMALA

Tel: +502 2362 0000
Therapist: Michelle Binford
Email:
info@dejadefumarfacil.com
Website: www.allencarr.com

HONG KONG

Email: info@easywayhongkong.com
Website: www.allencarr.com

HUNGARY

Seminars in Budapest and
12 other cities across Hungary
Tel: 06 80 624 426 (freephone) or
+36 20 580 9244
Therapist: Gábor Szász
Email: szasz.gabor@allencarr.hu
Website: www.allencarr.com

INDIA
Bangalore and Chennai

Tel: +91 (0)80 4154 0624
Therapist: Suresh Shottam
Email: info@
easywaytostopsmoking.co.in
Website: www.allencarr.com

IRAN

Please check website for details
Tehran and Mashhad
Website: www.allencarr.com

ISRAEL

Sessions held throughout Israel
Tel: +972 (0)3 6212525
Therapists: Orit Rozen and Team
Email: info@allencarr.co.il
Website: www.allencarr.com

ITALY

Sessions held throughout Italy
Tel/Fax: +39 (0)2 7060 2438
Therapists: Francesca Cesati and Team
Email: info@easywayitalia.com
Website: www.allencarr.com

JAPAN

Sessions held throughout Japan
www.allencarr.com

LEBANON
Tel: +961 1 791 5565
Therapist: Sadek El-Assaad
Email: info@AllenCarrEasyWay.me
Website: www.allencarr.com

MAURITIUS
Tel: +230 5727 5103
Therapist: Heidi Hoareau
Email: info@allencarr.mu
Website: www.allencarr.com

MEXICO
Sessions held throughout Mexico
Tel: +52 55 2623 0631
Therapists: Jorge Davo and Team
Email: info@allencarr-mexico.com
Website: www.allencarr.com

NETHERLANDS
Sessions held throughout the
Netherlands
Allen Carr's Easyway
'stoppen met roken'
Tel: +31 53 478 43 62/
+31 900 786 77 37
Email: info@allencarr.nl
Website: www.allencarr.com

NEW ZEALAND
North Island – Auckland
Tel: +64 (0) 800 848 028
Therapist: Natalie Clays and Team
Email: natalie@allencarr.co.nz
Website: www.allencarr.com

South Island – Wellington and Christchurch
Tel: +64 (0) 800 848 028
Therapist: Natalie Clays and Team
Email: natalie@allencarr.co.nz

NORWAY
Therapist: Laila Thorsen
Please check website for details
Website: www.allencarr.com

PERU
Lima
Tel: +511 637 7310
Therapist: Luis Loranca
Email: lloranca@
dejardefumaraltoque.com
Website: www.allencarr.com

POLAND
Sessions held throughout Poland
Tel: +48 (0)22 621 36 11
Therapist: Michael Spyrka
Email: info@allen-carr.pl
Website: www.allencarr.com

POLAND – Alcohol sessions
Tel: +48 71 307 32 37
Therapist: Maciej Kramarz
Email: mk@allen-carr.com.pl
Website: www.allencarr.com

PORTUGAL
Oporto
Tel: +351 22 9958698
Therapist: Ria Slof
Email:
info@comodeixardefumar.com
Website: www.allencarr.com

REPUBLIC OF IRELAND
Dublin
Tel: +353 (0)1 499 9010
Therapists: Paul Melvin & Jim McCreadie
Email: info@allencarr.ie

Website: www.allencarr.com

ROMANIA

Tel: +40 (0)7321 3 8383
Therapist: Cristina Nichita
Email: raspunsuri@allencarr.ro
Website: www.allencarr.com

RUSSIA

Allen Carr's Easyway to Stop
Smoking
Live Seminars & Online Video
Programme
Tel: +7 495 644 64 26
Freecall +7 (800) 250 6622
Therapist: Alexander Fomin
Email: info@allencarr.ru
Website: www.allencarr.com

Allen Carr's Easyway to Stop
Drinking
Live Seminars & Online Video
Programme
Tel: +8 (800) 302 80 68
+7 985 207 47 93
Therapist: Artem Kasyanov
Email: info@allencarrlife.ru
Website: www.allencarr.com

St Petersburg

Please check website for details
Website: www.allencarr.com

SERBIA
Belgrade

Tel: +381 (0)11 308 8686
Email: office@allencarr.co.rs
Website: www.allencarr.com

SINGAPORE

Tel: +65 62241450
Therapist: Pam Oei
Email: pam@allencarr.com.sg
Website: www.allencarr.com

SLOVENIA

Tel: +386 (0)40 77 61 77
Therapist: Grega Sever
Email: easyway@easyway.si
Website: www.allencarr.com

SOUTH AFRICA

Sessions held throughout South
Africa
National Booking Line:
0861 100 200
Head Office: 15 Draper Square,
Draper St, Claremont 7708, Cape
Town
Cape Town: Dr Charles Nel
Tel: +27 (0)21 851 5883
Mobile: 083 600 5555
Therapists: Dr Charles Nel,
Malcolm Robinson and Team
Email: easyway@allencarr.co.za
Website: www.allencarr.com

SOUTH KOREA
Seoul

Tel: +82 (0)70 4227 1862
Therapist: Yousung Cha
Email: master@allencarr.co.kr
Website: www.allencarr.com

SPAIN

Tel: +34 910 05 29 99
Therapist: Luis Loranca
Email: informes@AllenCarrOfficial.es
Website: www.allencarr.com

SWEDEN

Tel: +46 70 695 6850
Therapists: Nina Ljungqvist,
Renée Johansson
Email: info@easyway.se
Website: www.allencarr.com

SWITZERLAND

Sessions held throughout
Switzerland
Freephone: 0800RAUCHEN
(0800/728 2436)
Tel: +41 (0)52 383 3773
Fax: +41 (0)52 383 3774
Therapists: Cyrill Argast and Team
For sessions in Suisse Romand
and Svizzera Italiana:
Tel: 0800 386 387
Email: info@allen-carr.ch
Website: www.allencarr.com

TURKEY

Sessions held throughout Turkey
Tel: +90 212 358 5307
Therapist: Emre Üstünuçar
Email: info@allencarr.com.tr
Website: www.allencarr.com

UNITED ARAB EMIRATES
Dubai and Abu Dhabi

Tel: +97 56 693 4000
Therapist: Sadek El-Assaad
Email: info@AllenCarrEasyWay.me
Website: www.allencarr.com

OTHER ALLEN CARR PUBLICATIONS

Allen Carr's revolutionary Easyway method is available in a wide variety of formats, including digitally as audiobooks and ebooks, and has been successfully applied to a broad range of subjects. For more information about Easyway publications, please visit **shop.allencarr.com**

The Easy Way to Quit Smoking

The Easy Way to Quit Vaping

The Illustrated Easy Way to Stop Smoking

Allen Carr's Easy Way for Women to Quit Smoking

The Illustrated Easy Way for Women to Stop Smoking

Your Personal Stop Smoking Plan

Finally Free!

Smoking Sucks (Parent Guide with 16-page, pull-out comic)

The Little Book of Quitting Smoking

How to Be a Happy Nonsmoker

No More Ashtrays

The Only Way to Stop Smoking Permanently

How to Stop Your Child Smoking

The Easy Way to Control Alcohol

Allen Carr's Quit Drinking Without Willpower

Your Personal Stop Drinking Plan

Allen Carr's Easy Way for Women to Quit Drinking

The Illustrated Easy Way to Stop Drinking

No More Hangovers

The Easy Way to Mindfulness

Smart Phone Dumb Phone

Good Sugar Bad Sugar

The Easy Way to Quit Sugar

The Easy Way to Lose Weight

Allen Carr's Easy Way for Women to Lose Weight

No More Diets

The Easy Way to Stop Gambling

No More Gambling

No More Worrying

Get Out of Debt Now

No More Debt

No More Fear of Flying

The Easy Way to Quit Caffeine

Packing It In The Easy Way
(the autobiography)

Easyway publications are also available as **audiobooks**.
Visit **shop.allencarr.com** to find out more.

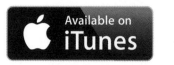 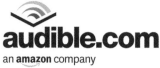